AGRICULTURE ISSUES AND POLICIES

ANTIBIOTIC USE IN U.S. LIVESTOCK PRODUCTION

ECONOMICS AND GUIDANCE ISSUES

AGRICULTURE ISSUES AND POLICIES

Additional books in this series can be found on Nova's website under the Series tab.

Additional e-books in this series can be found on Nova's website under the e-book tab.

AGRICULTURE ISSUES AND POLICIES

ANTIBIOTIC USE IN U.S. LIVESTOCK PRODUCTION

ECONOMICS AND GUIDANCE ISSUES

KARIN GREER
EDITOR

nova publishers
New York

Library of Congress Cataloging-in-Publication Data
ISBN: 978-1-63485-056-8

Published by Nova Science Publishers, Inc. † New York

CONTENTS

PREFACE

Farmers use antibiotics to treat, prevent, and control animal diseases and increase the productivity of animals and operations. However, there is concern that routine antibiotic use in livestock will contribute to antimicrobial-resistant pathogens, with repercussions for human and animal health. Given these concerns, pressure to limit antibiotic uses for purposes other than disease treatment is mounting. Changes in use will lead to a series of adjustments in animal agriculture as producers change production practices, with potential repercussions for prices and volumes in livestock markets. This book addresses the following questions: How widely are antibiotics used in the livestock industries? How could the current structure of the livestock industry influence the effects of restrictions on certain uses of antibiotics? How might the restriction of antibiotics affect production and costs at the animal and farm levels? How might those impacts affect production and prices in markets?

In: Antibiotic Use in U.S. Livestock Production ISBN: 978-1-63485-056-8
Editor: Karin Greer

Chapter 1

ECONOMICS OF ANTIBIOTIC USE IN U.S. LIVESTOCK PRODUCTION*

Stacy Sneeringer, James MacDonald, Nigel Key, William McBride and Ken Mathews

ABSTRACT

Farmers use antibiotics to treat, prevent, and control animal diseases and increase the productivity of animals and operations. However, there is concern that routine antibiotic use in livestock will contribute to antimicrobial-resistant pathogens, with repercussions for human and animal health. Given these concerns, pressure to limit antibiotic uses for purposes other than disease treatment is mounting. Changes in use will lead to a series of adjustments in animal agriculture as producers change production practices, with potential repercussions for prices and volumes in livestock markets. This report addresses the following questions: How widely are antibiotics used in the livestock industries? How could the current structure of the livestock industry influence the effects of restrictions on certain uses of antibiotics? How might the restriction of antibiotics affect production and costs at the animal and farm levels? How might those impacts affect production and prices in markets?

* This is an edited, reformatted and augmented version of Economic Research Report Number 200, issued by the U.S. Department of Agriculture, Economic Research Service, November 2015.

Keywords: antibiotics, livestock, United States, economics, prices, feed efficiency, production purposes, antimicrobials, growth promotion, policy analysis, disease prevention

WHAT IS THE ISSUE?

The animal agriculture sector is a major user of antibiotic drugs for disease treatment, disease control, disease prevention, and "production purposes" (such as growth promotion). Routine use of antibiotics—in humans or animals—can encourage antimicrobial resistance, which can lead to significant human and animal health risks. In 2013, the U.S. Food and Drug Administration (FDA) issued final guidance on voluntarily phasing out the use of medically important antibiotics (those important for therapeutic use in humans) for livestock production purposes.

This report addresses the following economic issues associated with the use of antibiotics in U.S. livestock agriculture:

1. How widely are antibiotics used in livestock production? What is the extent and purpose of use among different species and at different stages of production?
2. Are there discernible trends in the use of antibiotics for production and disease prevention by livestock producers?
3. How could the current structure of the livestock industry influence the effects of restrictions on antibiotics for production purposes?
4. How does the use of antibiotics for production purposes affect production and costs at the animal and farm levels?
5. How do the farm-level impacts of limiting production uses of antibiotics affect production and prices in markets?

WHAT DID THE STUDY FIND?

Extent of antibiotics for production-purpose and disease prevention use in livestock production - Administration of antibiotics for production or disease prevention uses in the live-stock sector is not universal and varies by species:

- **Hogs**. Between 2004 and 2009, the share of *finishing* hogs sold or removed from operations administering antibiotics to promote growth fell from 52 to 40 percent. The share from operations stating they did not know—or did not report—whether antibiotics were administered for growth promotion rose from 7 to 22 percent. The share of *nursery* hogs sold or removed from operations administering antibiotics for growth fell from 29 to 23 percent over 2004-2009. The share from operations stating that they did not know or report whether antibiotics were administered rose from 5 to 20 percent.
- **Broilers**. Between 2006 and 2011, the share of broilers raised *without* antibiotics except for disease treatment rose from 44 to 48 percent. The percentage of birds removed from operations reporting they did not know whether their birds were raised without antibiotics except for disease treatment rose from 29 to 32 percent.
- **Beef cattle**. While few beef/cow-calf operations use antibiotics for production purposes, they were fed to an estimated 49 percent of cattle at large-scale feedlots in 2011. In both 1994 and 2011, more than three-quarters of feedlots with at least 1,000 head provided antibiotics in feed or water, where the purpose is often growth promotion.
- **Dairy**. In 2006, an estimated one-fifth of dairy operations fed antibiotics to replacement heifers (milk cows that have not yet calved) for disease prevention. In 2007, 90.1 percent of dairy operations provided antibiotics for disease prevention.

Industry structure - Analysis of the structure of the pork, broiler, beef, and dairy subsectors suggests how limits on antibiotic use would affect the industries.

- Vertical integration—in which large firms control all or several parts of meat production, from feed mills to the retail level—influences which operations bear the costs of adjusting to restrictions on the use of antibiotics for production purposes. In many livestock industries, a majority of production is controlled by a few integrators who mostly determine feed formulations and use of antibiotics for production purposes; farmers may have little discretion in such uses of antibiotics.
- Livestock operations often specialize in specific phases of an animal's lifecycle. In certain stages, use of antibiotics for production purposes is more common and impactful. Hence, restrictions on the use of

antibiotics would have varying impacts on different types of farms and may have short-term effects on supply chains.

Effects of changes in use of antibiotics for production purposes on livestock producers and markets - Use of antibiotics for purposes other than disease treatment is associated with a 1- to 3-percent increase in productivity of a farm (not statistically distinguishable from no effect). Given this, we develop an estimate of the effects of restrictions on production uses of antibiotics on production, prices, and total revenue.

- For a given level of output, a 1- to 3- percent increase in the cost of production would lead to an increase of approximately 1 percent in wholesale prices and a drop in output of less than 1 percent.
- Producers using antibiotics for production purposes before restrictions are predicted to reduce production by 1 to 2 percent due to higher costs. They are predicted to see a decline of less than 1 percent in their value of production.
- Producers not using antibiotics for production purposes before restrictions are predicted to respond to higher prices by increasing production. Since their production costs for a given level of output do not increase due to restrictions, their total revenues increase.

HOW WAS THE STUDY CONDUCTED?

This report draws on data from the Agricultural Resource Management Survey (ARMS), jointly administered by the U.S. Department of Agriculture's National Agricultural Statistics Service (NASS) and Economic Research Service. The ARMS provides a representative sample of U.S. farming operations. The analysis also uses statistics from the National Animal Health Monitoring System conducted by the USDA's Animal and Plant Health Inspection Service and NASS.

The study modeled how restrictions in use of antibiotics for purposes other than disease treatment may affect market-level outcomes, including output and price.

INTRODUCTION

Antibiotics are used in livestock production to treat diseases in animals, to control the spread of disease among healthy animals in flocks and herds when diseased animals are present, to prevent disease even when no sick animals are present but there is a high likelihood of disease, and to increase animal productivity (so-called "production-purpose uses"). Improvements in productivity primarily include growing animals to market weight in less time and animals requiring less feed per unit of weight gain. For disease prevention and production purposes, antibiotics can be provided in subtherapeutic doses in feed or water (McEwan and Fedorka-Clay, 2002). Antibiotic use for disease prevention and production purposes is a common feature of modern U.S. livestock production, where animals are confined in barns, dry lots, or houses (see box, Definitions of "Production-purpose Uses" and "Antibiotic," p. 2).

Production-purpose antibiotics became widely used in U.S. livestock production in the 1970s because they reduced costs (CAST, 1981). Researchers as early as the 1940s discovered that animals that were fed low levels of antibiotics realized faster rates of growth and improved feed efficiency (Hays, 1991). This appears to operate through the antibiotic inhibition of normal microflora within the animal's gastrointestinal system, thereby enabling more energy to be expended for nutrient use and conversion to weight gain. If animals require less feed per unit of animal growth, producers are able to purchase fewer inputs per unit of output. Additionally, production-use antibiotics may reduce weight variability between animals, producing more uniform animals that are better suited to mechanized processing and that generate steadier income streams to farmers.

Regular use of antibiotics in humans or animals can lead to resistance among pathogens, and there is growing concern that widespread antibiotic use has led to the emergence of some organisms resistant to most or all antibiotics. The extent to which antibiotic use in livestock production contributes to human health problems is a matter of controversy. The U.S. Food and Drug Administration (FDA) has established that enough scientific evidence exists to support the agency's current restrictions on using medically important antibiotics for production purposes (U.S. FDA, 2012a). Other scientific and Government bodies posit a link between antibiotic use in livestock and human health risks (U.S. CDC, 2013; Infectious Diseases Society of America, 2010; WHO, 2012; Maves, 2009; Shea, 2004). While such a risk is present, its extent remains in question (Turnidge, 2004a; Chang et al., 2014).

In response to these concerns, public policy discussions have focused on the inappropriate use of antibiotics for human health and the use of production-purpose and disease-prevention antibiotics in animal agriculture, as well as on new antibiotic and vaccine approaches in both animal and human medicine. In 2006, the European Union (EU) banned the use of antibiotics for growth-promotion purposes, and subsequent bills have been introduced in the U.S. Congress (Johnson, 2011). In 2013, the FDA issued a final guidance document implementing voluntary plans to phase out the use of medically important[1] antibiotics in livestock for food production purposes (U.S. FDA, 2013). Another FDA proposal is to require that all medically important antibiotics require a veterinarian's prescription; at present, animal antibiotics are available over the counter without a prescription. Several major food retailers have placed restrictions on the use of antibiotics for production purposes by their meat suppliers (McDonald's, 2003; Weise, 2006; Pew Charitable Trusts, 2015), and there is growing consumer interest in products from animals raised without antibiotics (*Consumer Reports*, 2012). At the same time, there are concerns that poorly designed restrictions may pose new human and animal health risks and raise costs, without adequately addressing the risks of resistance.

Restricting use of antibiotics through Government intervention or voluntary actions is likely to have economic repercussions in animal agriculture. Producers may alter production practices, including the types of equipment and housing that they use, and they may seek out medicinal alternatives to antibiotics. They may adjust feed formulations or institute a number of alternative practices, such as bio-security measures and selective breeding. While these innovations may mitigate production losses due to lower antibiotic use, they will likely raise the costs of production, which will mean that less meat will be produced at a given price. As production volumes decline, prices will increase. Consumers may react to changes in meat prices and to perceptions about meat safety and quality, and retailers may adjust to changes in livestock production and consumer demand.

DEFINITIONS OF "PRODUCTION-PURPOSE USES" AND "ANTIBIOTICS"

Government documents, academic articles, and popular press refer to the different uses of antibiotics using a number of terms. In this report, we use the term "production-purpose uses" to refer to any antimicrobial use in livestock production for the purpose of productivity increases, such as faster growth and better feed efficiency (less feed per unit of weight gain). Thus, our definition depends on purpose, not on amount of antibiotic used. Purpose of use is specific to species, disease, and type of antibiotic and is listed on drug labels. Our selection of terms corresponds to recent FDA guidance documents (FDA, 2012a). In this report we also occasionally make use of other terms to refer to antibiotic use. Antibiotics are used for four main purposes in livestock production: (1) Disease treatment; (2) Disease control (metaphylatic); (3) Disease prevention (prophylactic); and (4) Production. Other terms used in the literature and the purposes they cover are:

- "Subtherapeutic" can refer to 3 or 4, and is often used to only refer to 4.
- "Nontherapeutic" can refer to 2, 3, or 4, but is often used to refer to only 3 or 4.
- "Antimicrobial growth promotion" (AGP) is a type of 4.

We use these alternative terms most frequently when describing documents that use them.

While our focus in much of the report is production uses of antibiotics, we also pay particular attention to prophylactic (disease prevention) uses, for two reasons:

1. The policy dialogue in the United States and other countries includes both production and prophylactic uses. While recent FDA actions have focused on production uses, there are calls in the United States to also restrict prophylactic uses (Lawrence, 2012; Mellon, 2013; WHO, 2000).

Certain European countries have also placed limitations on prophylactic uses of antibiotics, based on concerns that producers will switch from production to prevention use when production use is restricted (Jensen and Hayes, 2014; Levy, 2014).

2. The survey data from which we draw statistics do not always distinguish between production and prophylactic uses. For example, in the Agricultural and Resource Management Surveys (ARMS) broiler questionnaires, respondents are asked if they raised birds without antibiotics in their feed or water unless the birds were sick. Hence, prophylactic uses, occurring when disease is possible but not yet evident, are not distinguished from production uses in the survey.

The term "antibiotics" also warrants clarification, particularly in its relation to "antimicrobials" and "anti-bacterials." Technically, antimicrobials encompass antibacterials, which encompass antibiotics. Hence, all antibiotics are antimicrobials, but not all antimicrobials are antibiotics. Despite these differences, the terms "antimicrobials" and "antibiotics" are often used interchangeably. As a recent FDA document notes:

> "The term 'antimicrobials' refers broadly to drugs with activity against a variety of microorganisms including bacteria, viruses, fungi, and parasites. Antimicrobial drugs that have specific activity against bacteria are referred to as antibacterial or antibiotic drugs. However, the broader term 'antimicrobial,' commonly used in reference to drugs with activity against bacteria, is used … interchangeably with the terms antibacterial or antibiotic" (U.S. FDA, 2012a, p. 4).

In this report, we generally use the term "antibiotics" interchangeably with "antimicrobials." Confusion surrounds ionophores and coccidiostats, which are antimicrobials used in livestock production but not in human medicine. The USDA's Food Safety and Inspection Service (FSIS) defines ionophores to be antibiotics for label claims. Where possible, we specify a distinction between antibiotics exclusive of ionophores and coccidiostats.

How restrictions will affect the different livestock industries will depend in part on how these industries are structured. Industries with a higher degree of concentration and fewer decision makers will be able to have greater immediate impact on use of antibiotics than industries with more entities making decisions about feed formulations. If use of antibiotics for production purposes has a larger impact on certain stages of the animal life-cycle, restrictions on such use may disrupt supply chains in industries that divide the lifecycle portions among operations, at least in the short term.

The impact of restrictions on use of antibiotics will also depend on how widely they are used and how they are used among different species and stages of production. Current policies are phasing out production uses of antibiotics that are important in human medicine; livestock industries relying on such antibiotics may encounter more compliance difficulties than industries that use antibiotics specific to animal medicine (such as antimicrobials like ionophores or coccidiostats). If production-purpose antibiotics are not used universally, restrictions on use will have less impact on industries as a whole and on market outcomes.

The effect of production-purpose antibiotic restrictions on market quantities and prices will depend on the extent of antibiotic use and the farm-level impacts of use. If use is limited and productivity effects are small, then effects on overall production and price changes may be small. The inverse is true as well. Producers not using antibiotics for production purposes may even enjoy higher returns if restrictions also create higher prices for meat and consumers do not distinguish between products raised with and without production-purpose antibiotics.

Antibiotic Uses in Livestock Production

Antibiotics are used in livestock production for four main purposes, and the route of administration is often specific to the purpose (McEwen and Fedorka-Clay, 2002):

- To treat animals that fall ill (disease treatment).
- To prevent illness in healthy animals when diseased animals are present (metaphylactic uses or disease control). If some animals become ill, the rest of the animals in a pen or barn may receive a dose of antibiotics to prevent the illness from spreading. The treatment may also provide protection from animals already infected but not yet showing symptoms.
- To prevent disease in healthy animals when no animals display signs of disease (prophylactic uses or disease prevention). Prophylactic uses of antibiotics include administering antibiotics to all animals in a group setting where there is high risk of a disease outbreak. Generally,

drugs are administered to prevent a specific disease that has a high likelihood of occurring.

- To promote faster or more efficient livestock growth (production purposes). Nutrition studies in the 1940s and 50s demonstrated that antibiotics could lead to faster growth and improved conversion of feed to weight gain, and antibiotics have been administered for growth promotion since then (CAST, 1981). Antibiotics are thought to promote animal growth through their effects on gut microflora. Bacterial species in the gut compete with the host for nutrients and can therefore absorb some of the nutrients provided to animals in feed and water, preventing them from contributing to the animal's weight gain. Antibiotics appear to promote growth by suppressing those bacteria (Dibner and Richards, 2005). Preventive use of antibiotics may also enable growth promotion or increases in feed efficiency.

In addition to promoting growth and increasing feed efficiency, antibiotic use may result in less variability in weight and can also have reproductive benefits. For production purposes, antibiotics are administered at subtherapeutic levels, generally via medicated feed. Antibiotics fed at production-purpose doses may also prevent disease.

The overlap between the dosage levels and types of antibiotics used for disease prevention and production purposes has led to controversy over what uses would be limited under various policies. Many proposed policies, including the 2013 guidance document adopted by the FDA, aim to reduce the use of antibiotics for production purposes. There is concern that even if antibiotics were not labeled for growth promotion, producers could continue to feed allowable, disease-preventing antibiotics at a growth-promotion level (U.S. GAO, 2011).

Public Health Concerns with Antibiotic Use in Livestock Production

There are two main areas of concern about the human health effects of antibiotic use in livestock production:

- **Antibiotic residues in food products,** which may cause allergic reactions and digestive problems in humans, were the focus of early regulation of antibiotics in food animals (NRC, 1999). The FDA therefore established minimum intervals between the last dose of antimicrobials and the time of slaughter to prevent such residues in meat (U.S. FDA, 2014a).

- **The threat of drug-resistant bacteria.** Studies have reported the appearance of drug-resistant bacteria in food animals shortly after antibiotic use in production began (Dibner and Richards, 2005), though recent studies have shown antibiotic resistance in the natural environment predates production uses (Bhullar et al., 2012).

Drug-resistant bacteria in animals may harm human health via three main routes of transmission. First, humans may consume or otherwise come in contact with food that is contaminated with drug-resistant bacteria, which may occur at many processing points, including sale, storage, and preparation. Second, humans may come in contact with resistant bacteria via live farm animals, manure, or shed material such as feathers. Drug-resistant bacteria may infect producers, processing- facility workers, or others who live or work on farms. Third, infected people can then transmit illness to others.

Tracking the actual transmission of antimicrobial-resistant diseases due to production-purpose antibiotics between animals and humans is difficult, involving several steps. First, researchers must find an association between the proliferation and persistence of resistant bacteria in animals from production-purpose doses of antimicrobial drugs. Second, researchers must show the presence of resistant pathogens in animals or animal products exposed to production-purpose levels of antibiotics. Third, studies must link the transmission of these pathogens to humans. Finally, researchers must diagnose human diseases caused by these pathogens. Despite the difficulty in making all of these linkages, studies that trace human infections by drug-resistant pathogens to animal sources do exist (see Harrison et al., 2013; Morley et al., 2011; Cohen and Tauxe, 1986; Holmberg, Wells, and Cohen, 1984), but not without caveats and inconsistencies (e.g., Mather et al., 2013; Price et al., 2012).

While antibiotics fed to livestock have been linked to human health risks, the extent of these risks remains a matter of debate. Public health advocacy groups calculate that 80 percent of the antibiotics sold in the United States go to livestock (Loglisci, 2010). However, the FDA contends that this figure is problematic for a number of reasons and warns against direct comparisons of amounts of antibiotics sold for human versus animal consumption (U.S. FDA, 2012c). Industry groups also argue that most of the antibiotics used in livestock production are not critical to treating human illnesses (Raymond, 2013). Other authors cite research showing that even antibiotics not used in human medicine may lead to the development of bacteria resistant to antibiotics necessary to treat human illness (Consumers Union, undated). A livestock industry-funded study argues that the effect of antibiotic use for

Table 1. Potential effects of use of antibiotics for production and disease prevention purposes at the animal, farm, and market levels of aggregation

Level of aggregation Factor	Possible effects of antibiotics for production and disease prevention uses
Animal-level factors	
Average daily gain	Use may increase the rate of daily gain, which allows animals to reach market weight in less time.
Feed efficiency (amount of feed required per amount of gain)	Use may lower the amount of feed required per unit of weight gain, allowing less feed to be used.
Mortality rate of young animals	Use may lead to lowered mortality rate of young animals.
Morbidity (illness rates)	Use may lower certain types of illness.
Live pigs born per litter	Use may increase the animals born per litter.
Percentage of breeding pigs that farrowed	Use may increase the percentage of inseminated breeding pigs that give birth.
Variability in product	Use may reduce variation between animals, making products more uniform.
Farm-level factors	
Veterinary costs	Use may decrease veterinary costs as it may play a role in disease prevention.
Costs of antibiotics used for production or disease prevention uses	Use will increase the total cost of antibiotics used for production or disease prevention uses.
Costs of antibiotics for disease treatment	Use for production or disease prevention purposes may decrease costs for disease treatment.
Feed costs	Use may lower feed costs due to greater feed efficiency.
Labor costs	Operators may spend less time caring for ill animals, decreasing labor costs.
Costs of biosecurity measures	Producers may use antibiotics for disease prevention and production purposes instead of biosecurity measures; hence, use may be linked to lower costs of these other practices.
Variability in revenues	A decrease in the variability of the product may decrease market-level penalties for animals outside a weight range for mechanized processing.
Economies of scale	Use may reduce the amount of space needed per animal, so that more animals can be raised in the same area.
Market-level factors	
Total cost of production	Use may reduce the total cost of production.
Total quantity of meat and livestock products produced	If use lowers total costs of production, producers can produce more output per unit of input.
Meat and livestock product prices	If use lowers the total cost of production and producers produce more output per unit of input, prices will fall.

Revenue from selling meat or livestock products	In the short term, early adopters of antibiotics for disease prevention or production purposes may receive profits related to use. As use becomes common, quantity will increase and prices will fall, leading to zero revenue related to use (profits).
Demand for meat	Reduction of use for disease prevention or production purposes may lead to greater demand for meat. If use leads to lower prices, this may also increase demand for meat.
U.S. exports of meat and livestock products	Use may reduce exports if importing countries want meat raised sans antibiotics for disease prevention or production purposes. Use may increase exports if it enables lower U.S. meat prices.

Source: USDA, Economic Research Service.

growth promotion is likely to have little clinical significance for humans (Phillips et al., 2004). However, this study has been critiqued as not accurately representing all published research (Turnidge, 2004a and 2004b). At present, the extent to which antibiotic use in livestock production contributes to human health problems is unknown, and thus the size of the benefits from restricting use is also unknown.

Economic Aspects of Production-Purpose Uses of Antibiotics in Livestock Production

Antibiotic use for production purposes in the U.S. livestock industry has economic ramifications at three levels: the farm animal, the farm, and the market (Table 1). Production uses of antibiotics can have a number of impacts on animal productivity, notably growth and feed efficiency (more meat produced per unit of feed).

Using antibiotics for production purposes can reduce input costs; if animals can gain the same amount of weight with less feed, then more output can be produced per dollar of input. Indirectly, antibiotics used for production purposes or disease prevention may influence the scale and type of production; if antibiotics reduce the prevalence of disease, then more animals can be raised per square foot. If antibiotic use is reduced, producers are likely to adjust production processes. They may provide more feed to reach production targets, but they may also use other animal drugs or vaccines, alter sanitation practices, or modify housing environments through capital investments. Such adjustments affect the financial impacts of reducing antibiotic use and may also affect animal health and environmental outcomes.

If use of antibiotics for production purposes allows ***farmers*** to produce more output per unit of input, then this may lower prices and increase supply. Because antibiotics affect feed efficiency, reducing their use may increase demand for feed, with ramifications for grain markets. To the extent that restrictions on production-purpose antibiotics increase production costs, the United States may become less competitive in meat export markets.

Market-level effects of production-purpose antibiotics occur on both the production and demand side. Consumer awareness of antibiotic use in livestock production has increased. One indication of the growing demand for products raised with limited antibiotic use is a *Consumer Reports* 2012 survey finding that 86 percent of consumers would like the ability to buy meat raised without antibiotics at their local supermarket (*Consumer Reports*, 2012). This survey of 1,000 U.S. residents found that over 60 percent would be willing to pay an additional $0.05 per pound for meat raised without antibiotics, and 37 percent were willing to pay an additional dollar per pound.[2] A majority of respondents stated they were concerned about widespread use of antibiotics in animal feed and possible effects on antibiotic-resistant viruses.

The growing organic market is another indicator of burgeoning demand for products raised without antibiotics. Products labeled as organic by the USDA must be produced without antibiotics fed or administered to the animal at any point in its life. Sales of foods labeled organic have risen from $11 billion in 2004 to approximately $32 billion in 2013 (Osteen et al., 2012; Greene, 2014). However, organics still constitute a small minority of livestock production. In addition, the organic label refers to many attributes of the product, not just the absence of antibiotics used in production. Hence, the increased production and sales of organic products may reflect demand for these other attributes.

The demands of individual consumers can also affect the practices of retailers. The Consumer Reports study found that of the 13 largest grocery retailers (by sales), 11 offered either meat labeled as organic or raised without antibiotics (2012). Fast-food companies have also begun demanding meat with fewer antibiotics. In 2003, the McDonald's Corporation issued a statement that it would use only meat raised without antibiotics for growth promotion (McDonald's, 2003);[3] the U.S. branch of the corporation reiterated its commitment to sourcing antibiotic-free meat in 2015 (McDonald's, 2015). By early 2006, several media reports indicated that four major chicken companies had phased out such antibiotic uses (Weise, 2006). Many major retailers and food service providers have also taken steps to reduce their demand for meat raised with antibiotics (Pew Charitable Trusts, 2015).

Alternatives to Uses of Antibiotics for Production Purposes and Disease Prevention in Livestock Production

Many methods and substitutes have been investigated for reducing the use of antibiotics in animal husbandry. Generally, these alternatives can be divided into those used to prevent disease and those used for growth promotion. These two goals may overlap, as animals that are not fighting disease may grow faster or display greater feed efficiency when they are fed antibiotics for disease prevention.

Management practices can both prevent disease and its transmission and enhance animal productivity (Smith, 2011). Improving living conditions for animals can lead to less stress and hence better immunity. Stress reduction can occur through better heat, humidity, and ventilation management, limiting the introduction of new pen mates, and increasing space per animal (NRC, 1999). Heat stress can be reduced through evaporative cooling and design changes in production buildings.

Measures to promote biosecurity (the protection of agricultural animals from any type of infectious agent) can also reduce the incidence of disease at production facilities, reducing the need for antibiotics. One biosecurity measure is exclusion of potential pathogen carriers from the premises, including wild animals, domestic pets, and workers not essential to the operation. Other measures include prompt removal of dead animals, increased hygiene within production facilities, and locating barns away from potential sources of infection (NRC, 1999).

Optimizing nutrition can also encourage animal immunity. High-energy food rations can be fed to animals to increase growth and to reduce the effects of stressors. Adapting nutrients in feed to specific stages of growth can also boost immunity. In addition, supplementation with specific micro-nutrients (vitamins and minerals) has been shown to reduce disease (NRC, 1999).

As mentioned, the effect of antibiotics on growth promotion is thought to be related to the gut micro-flora. Hence, alternatives to antibiotics often focus on impacting the gut ecosystem. One strategy is to discourage the proliferation of undesirable organisms in the animals' digestive systems by encouraging beneficial microorganisms in the gut (in contrast to antibiotics, which are believed to reduce harmful organisms). This strategy includes feeding enzymes, organic acids, prebiotics, probiotics, and immune modulators (Choct, 2001; Doyle, 2001).

A number of other methods can be used to promote growth and prevent disease (Oliver and Wells, 2013; Nemechek et al., 2013). Animals that are disease resistant can be selectively bred. Vaccinations can prevent some diseases, reducing the need for antibiotics. These methods may cost more than antibiotics. Replacing antibiotics used for production purposes or disease prevention may thus require more labor, capital, or material on farms, raising production costs.

U.S. and European Policy Instruments

Several U.S. Government agencies oversee the use of antibiotics in livestock production, including the FDA, the USDA, and the U.S. Centers for Disease Control and Prevention (CDC). The variety of the programs offers several layers of protection to guard the public health from antibiotic residues and antimicrobial resistance.

FDA Approval Process for Antibiotics Used in Food Animal Production

The FDA requires a rigorous multistep approval process for any antimicrobial to be used in livestock production. Once the antimicrobial drug sponsor has tested the drug for safety and effectiveness, the FDA's Center for Veterinary Medicine (CVM) reviews the sponsor's testing results and decides whether the approval requirements are met. If they are, the sponsor submits an application for approval to CVM, including all information about the drug and the proposed label. The sponsor can legally sell the antimicrobial drug if, upon review, the CVM agrees that the drug is safe and effective (U.S. FDA, 2014a).

As part of its approval for any antibiotic used in livestock production, the FDA establishes minimum withdrawal periods between the last use of the antibiotic and slaughter. The withdrawal time allows for the drug (or parts of the drug) to fall below the tolerance level deemed appropriate for human consumption. If the withdrawal time is observed, food products made from the treated animal are considered safe for people to eat (U.S. FDA, 2014a).

Monitoring Antibiotic Residues and Antimicrobial Resistance in Meat and Dairy Products

USDA's Food Safety and Inspection Service (FSIS) monitors animal products at slaughter facilities and U.S. ports of entry to test antibiotic residue levels (as well as other substances) in meat samples. Examining just the domestic meat, in 2011 FSIS tested 5,006 samples for antibiotic residues and found 8 violations (an overall rate of 0.16 percent among scheduled samples) (USDA, FSIS, 2013). Carcasses found with residue violations may be partly or entirely condemned. Producers of meat with violations are reported in the publicly available FSIS Residue Violation Information System.

The FDA also has primary responsibility for monitoring antibiotic residues in milk. Monitoring is carried out by State regulatory agencies, acting under contracts with the FDA, through the Grade "A" Milk Pasteurized Milk Ordinance (PMO). The Grade "A" PMO, whose primary purpose is to initiate and maintain effective programs for the prevention of milk-borne disease, was developed in 1924 as the Standard Milk Ordinance and was most recently revised in 2011 (U.S. FDA, 2011). Monitoring occurs at several points along the supply chain from dairy to consumer. If cows have been treated with antibiotics, they must undergo a withdrawal period before they can be milked again to generate products for human consumption in order to prevent residues in milk. Dairy processors engage in extensive sampling and testing of milk and cows to manage production, set compensation, meet public health requirements, and detect and manage animal diseases on the farm. Milk from cows is collected in specialized tankers at dairy operations, either daily or every other day. Milk samples are taken from each tanker arriving at a processing plant, and if a sample tests positive for antibiotics, the entire tank must be dumped, entailing a financial cost to the producer. Specialized labs, supported by an extensive reporting and sample transportation system, perform this testing.

The FSIS also tests for antimicrobial-resistant bacteria under the National Antimicrobial Resistance Monitoring System's (NARMS) Enteric Bacteria program, originally established in 1996 (U.S. FDA, 2014b). The main purpose of the program is to serve as a safety monitoring system for antibiotics approved by the FDA, with the overarching goal of helping to preserve the effectiveness of medically important antimicrobial drugs used in food-producing animals. The FDA has used information gathered through NARMS to withdraw approval for certain antibiotics and to write guidance for the industry on the judicious use of antibiotics in livestock.

The NARMS program includes three branches, which monitor humans, retail meat, and food animals. Monitoring of human samples is carried out by the CDC, while monitoring of retail meat is performed by the FDA's Center for Veterinary Medicine (CVM) in conjunction with the CDC. To monitor food animals, isolates collected from animal products at slaughter are tested for resistance to 17 antibiotics. Figure 1 shows that for 4 animal groups, the percentage of samples resistant to none of the 17 antibiotics tested was either declining or remaining level between 1999 and 2010.

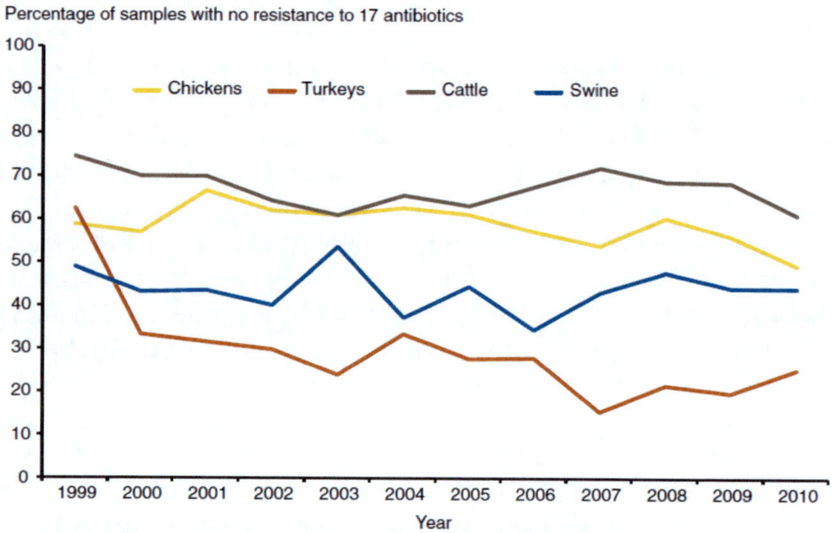

Source: National Antimicrobial Resistance Monitoring System.

Figure 1. Percentage of nontyphoidal salmonella isolates from food animals with no resistance to 17 antibiotics, 1999-2010, by type of food animal.

Labeling Antibiotic Use in Meat and Dairy Products

USDA's FSIS also develops and implements regulations and policies to ensure that meat, poultry, and egg-product labeling is truthful and not misleading. Under the 1906 Federal Meat Inspection Act and the 1957 Poultry Products Inspection Act, the labels of meat and poultry products must be approved by the U.S. Secretary of Agriculture, who has delegated this authority to FSIS, before these products can enter commerce.

FSIS reviews labeling regarding nutrition or health claims, as well as claims that the product is free of specified substances. Increasingly, though,

FSIS is asked to review and approve label claims regarding how animals are raised, such as "organic," "free-range," "cage-free," or "raised without antibiotics."

The Consumer Reports survey noted above indicates that many consumers would place a high value on products raised without antibiotics and would be willing to pay more for such products. Effective labeling could therefore put market forces behind efforts to reduce antibiotic use in livestock production; if firms that incur higher costs to produce animals without antibiotics were able to realize higher prices and substantial sales volumes, profit motives could induce shifts away from production practices that rely heavily on antibiotics. Accurate and truthful labeling is essential to maintaining the consumer confidence that would allow such a market to develop.

In evaluating claims about how animals are raised, FSIS faces several challenges. The agency must ascertain the precise meaning of the claim, as understood by consumers; it must develop processes to verify claims; and, given the perceived value of such claims, it must have a means to identify unapproved label claims.

Verifying claims of how animals are raised can be more difficult than claims regarding nutrition and ingredients, which can be supported with data on a product's composition and tested in laboratory settings. Meat and poultry products do not provide evidence of how animals were raised, so laboratory tests are of no help, and the agency does not have the resources to perform inspections of farms or ranches, even if products could be traced back to them.

U.S. Policy Actions to Reduce Use of Antibiotics for Production Purposes in Livestock Production

In the United States, the FDA first approved use of certain antibiotics in livestock feed in 1951 but proposed ending uses of antibiotics for production purposes in livestock production beginning in the 1970s. In 1970, the FDA published a task force study that concluded that long-term use of antibiotics in food-producing animals might pose a threat to human health. The task force recommended that antibiotics used in human medicine that failed to meet certain guidelines be prohibited for production use in dairy and meat animals. It also recommended that antibiotics be administered only by a veterinarian or with a veterinarian's prescription (U.S. FDA, 2012a).

As a result of the 1970 FDA report, antibiotic drug sponsors were required to submit study results by 1975 demonstrating that their products did not pose a threat to human health. In 1977, the FDA moved to withdraw penicillin and tetracycline for subtherapeutic use in animal feed. However, Congress directed the FDA to wait on the proposed withdrawal until further study could be conducted.

To carry out further study, the FDA first contracted with the National Academy of Science (NAS) to examine research published to date on the association between human health and subtherapeutic use of penicillin and tetracycline in animal feed. The NAS issued its report in 1980, which noted that the epidemiologic studies of the human health effects of antibiotic use in animal production were few and involved small samples of subjects and short time periods. The study concluded that the available data could neither prove nor disprove that antibiotic use in animals led to human health hazards and suggested that definitive studies to answer this question might not even be possible (U.S. FDA, 2012a).

The FDA continued to support research into the safety of subtherapeutic antibiotic use (Institute of Medicine, 1988; Seattle King County Department of Public Health, 1984). Over the next three decades, additional studies provided overviews of the existing research that associated antimicrobial use in livestock and human disease resistance (World Health Organization, 1997; National Research Council, 1999; U.S. GAO, 1999; European Agency for the Evaluation of Medicinal Products, 1999; World Health Organization, 2002; Institute of Medicine, 2003).

In 2003, the FDA issued guidance to pharmaceutical companies to include a risk assessment during the preapproval evaluation for any *new* antibiotics to be used in livestock agriculture. However, this did not apply to the majority of antibiotics used in meat production, which were approved for use prior to 2003. To mitigate the use of antibiotics approved before 2003, the FDA would need to withdraw agency approval for the specific use of a drug. This is a lengthy and challenging process. For example, the FDA took approximately 5 years to withdraw approval for enrofloxacin, a type of fluoroquinolone, based on evidence of increasing resistance in humans and animals (U.S. GAO, 2011). The drug was finally withdrawn from use in poultry production in 2005.

Instead of attempting to initiate formal withdrawal proceedings on numerous individual antibiotics, in June of 2010 the FDA released a draft of voluntary guidelines requesting that all medically important antibiotics in livestock be limited to disease treatment, control, or prevention purposes and stating that the antibiotics would require veterinary oversight in use. Following the release of these voluntary guidelines, in late 2011 the FDA withdrew its

1977 proposal to end approval for penicillin and tetracycline for subtherapeutic use in animal feed (this proposal was never adopted). The FDA argued that it would instead rely on voluntary responses by the industry.

In 2011, the FDA released draft guidance recommending strategies to implement "judicious use" of antimicrobial drugs in livestock production. In congressional testimony, the principal deputy commissioner stated that that the "FDA concludes that the overall weight of evidence to date supports the conclusion that using medically important antimicrobial drugs for production purposes is not in the interest of protecting and promoting the public health" (Sharfstein, 2010, p. 49). In the same hearing, a representative from the CDC stated, "There is unequivocal and compelling evidence that the use of antibiotics in animals leads to the development of drug-resistant bacteria that have adverse impacts on human public health" (Khan, 2010, p. 58).

In 2012, FDA Guidance for Industry #209 was finalized. It describes the overall policy that focuses on the "judicious use" of antibiotics in livestock production and aims to limit medically important antibiotic use to "those uses that are considered necessary for assuring animal health" and "that include veterinary oversight or consultation" (U.S. FDA, 2012a, pp. 21-22). Hence, "judicious use" excludes medically important antibiotics from use to promote growth or improve feed efficiency because "unlike other uses of those drugs in animals (e.g., for the treatment, control, and prevention of disease), these 'production uses' are not intended to manage specific disease that may be ongoing or at risk of occurring" (U.S. FDA, 2012a, p. 4). Historically, most medicated feeds could be purchased over the counter and did not require veterinary oversight.

In 2013, the FDA released a second guidance document (#213) to provide more detailed information to pharmaceutical manufacturers on how to align their medically important antimicrobial products that were approved for use in the feed or water of food-producing animals with Guidance #209, which meant withdrawing production uses and requiring that any remaining over-the-counter uses have veterinary oversight (U.S. FDA, 2013). As of June 2014, all 26 companies producing antibiotics used in livestock feed had agreed to the FDA's request (U.S. FDA, 2014c).

Congressional legislators have also repeatedly proposed bills to limit use of antibiotics in livestock agriculture. For example, the Preservation of Antibiotics for Medical Treatment Act (PAMTA) was first proposed in 2007 and has been reintroduced in every subsequent Congress. This legislation would in effect eliminate both disease prevention and production uses in livestock production of antibiotics used in human medicine. A number of consumer organizations, as well as the American Medical Association, support the adoption of PAMTA.

European Policies for Reducing Uses of Antibiotics for Production Purposes and Disease Prevention in Livestock Production

European lawmaking related to antibiotics used for production or disease prevention purposes has followed a different trajectory from that of the United States. In 1969, the "Swann Report" to the British Parliament, formally a report from the Joint Committee on the Use of Antibiotics in Animal Husbandry and Veterinary Medicine headed by Dr. M. M. Swann, suggested that increasing antibiotic resistance among humans was related to antibiotic use in livestock. The Swann Committee recommended banning the feeding of antibiotics at subtherapeutic levels to animals based on this concern.

Following publication of the Swann Report, in the early 1970s, the United Kingdom banned the use of penicillin and tetracycline as growth promoters (Hughes and Heritage, 2004). Other European countries began banning specific antibiotics as livestock growth promoters in the 1980s and 1990s. In 1986, Sweden was the first country to ban all antimicrobial growth promoters (Aarestrup, 2003). Norway banned over-the-counter antibiotics in feed in 1992; Finland did so in 1996, followed by Poland and Switzerland in 1999 (Hayes et al., 1999). In 1997, the Commission of the European Union banned avoparcin for use in livestock feed in all member States; it banned the use of several other antibiotics for production purposes in 1999. An EU ban on all antibiotics as growth promoters went into effect in 2006.

Denmark's experiences with reducing production and disease prevention uses of antibiotics have been well studied. In 1995, the country banned avoparcin and followed suit with virginiamycin in 1998. The Danish cattle and broiler industries voluntarily discontinued use of all antimicrobial growth promoters in 1998; the swine industry ended growth-promoting antimicrobial use in finishing hogs in 1998 and in all hogs in 1999 (WHO, 2002). Denmark also limited the ability for veterinarians to profit from sales of antibiotics and increased monitoring of prescriptions (Jensen and Hayes, 2014). In 2010, the Danish Government adopted a "Yellow Card" scheme based on prescription monitoring: producers that used more than a specific amount of antibiotic per pig were issued a warning. If producers failed to lower their use, they faced additional oversight at their own expense and eventually would be forced to either reduce use or decrease the herd size (Jensen and Hayes, 2014).

Before Denmark's ban fully took place, the Danish Ministry of Food and Agriculture also put in place the Integrated Antimicrobial Resistance Monitoring and Research Programme (DANMAP), which tallies antimicrobial usage in both livestock and people. Based in part on thorough data collection, researchers have been able to study the effects of Denmark's ban on antibiotic use as well as animal productivity, morbidity, and mortality.

One concern with a ban eliminating use of antibiotics for growth promotion is that it would lead to more disease treatment use. Figure 2 shows the amount of antimicrobial agents (in kilograms) prescribed for all types of animals in Denmark between 1990 and 2012. The dates of the bans and the voluntary stoppages are shown, as are the amounts used for growth promotion and other use. While the total amount of antimicrobials used for purposes other than growth promotion has indeed grown since the original 1995 ban, the total amount in 2012 is still less than pre-ban levels. Part of this rise in uses other than growth promotion is attributable to increasing pork production (shown on the figure). In 2012, pigs accounted for over three-quarters of antimicrobial agents consumed in Denmark (DANMAP, 2012).

Figure 2 shows the total amount of antibiotics used in Danish livestock, but it does not account for the dosage or amount of active ingredients, which could change over time and impact the total amount of antimicrobials used. In a study using 120 Danish farrow-to-finish swine farms from 1998 to 2000, the number of doses of antimicrobials *increased* in weaner pigs after the ban (WHO 2002). The "animal daily dose" (ADD) went from 0.8 ADD per pig-month before the ban to 1.5 ADD per pig-month after the ban (WHO, 2002, p. 19). The increase remained at this higher level for 12 months after the ban. In finisher pigs, the ADD increased from 0.2 per pig-month prior to the ban to 0.4 ADD per pig-month after the ban. However, the frequency returned to pre-ban levels within 1 year after the ban (WHO, 2002, p. 19). There is further examination of changes in livestock outcomes associated with European bans in later sections and in Appendix A.

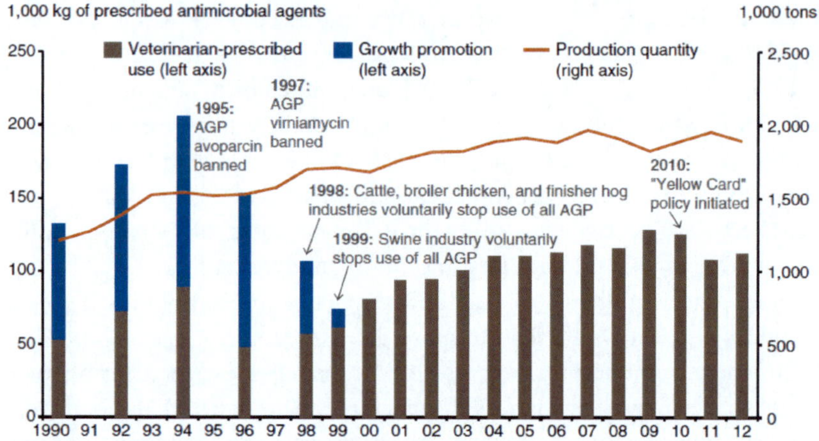

Sources: The Danish Integrated Antimicrobial Resistance Monitoring and Research Programme 1999 and 2010, 2011, and 2012. Data on growth promotion amounts not collected in 1991, 1993, 1995, and 1997. Production quantity data is from the United Nations Food and Agriculture Organization (FAOSTAT), Statistical Databases: http://faostat.fao.org/site/569/default.aspx#ancor. "AGP" refers to "antimicrobial growth promoter."

Figure 2. Consumption of antimicrobial agent use in all types of animals in Denmark and production of pork, 1990-2012, with dates of policy actions.

ANTIBIOTIC USE IN THE HOG, BROILER, BEEF, AND DAIRY INDUSTRIES

Survey Data on Antibiotics Used in the U.S. Livestock Industry

This report uses data and statistics from two main sources, the Agricultural and Resource Management Survey (ARMS) and the NAHMS.

Agricultural and Resource Management Survey (ARMS)

The ARMS is an annual, nationally representative survey of U.S. farms administered jointly by USDA's Economic Research Service (ERS) and National Agricultural Statistics Service (NASS). Used primarily to collect information on farm finances, production practices, and resource use, the ARMS generally focuses on one to three commodities each year, including livestock. Surveys of commodities are rotated so that data are gathered on a specific crop or type of livestock every 5 to 6 years. Some livestock surveys have included questions on antibiotic use. The ARMS is designed to be representative of U.S. agriculture, and the livestock versions represent commercial producers in States comprising at least 90 percent of production. Table 2 shows the years, commodities, and basic characteristics of the ARMS surveys used in this study.

Table 2. Characteristics of ARMS surveys used in this report

Survey	Targeted population	Percentage of U.S. animals covered	Percentage of U.S. operations covered	States included
ARMS – Hogs – 2004	Operations with 25 or more hogs onsite at any time during the year	91% of ending-year hog inventory[1]	59% of operations with hogs[2]	AR, CO, GA, IL, IN, IA, KS, KY, MI, MN, MO, NE, NC, OH, OK, PA, SD, VA, WI
ARMS – Hogs – 2009	Operations with 25 or more hogs onsite at any time during the year	94% of ending-year hog inventory[1]	34% of hog operations[2]	AR, CO, GA, IL, IN, IA, KS, KY, MI, MN, MO, NE, NC, OH, OK, PA, SD, VA, WI
ARMS – Broilers – 2006	Operations that produced broilers for meat and had at least 1,000 broilers onsite at any time during the year	98% of broiler production[3]	2006 ARMS included 17,183 growers compared with 16,046 in 2007[4]	AL, AR, CA, DE, GA,KY, LA, MD, MS, MO, NC, OK, PA, SC, TN, TX, VA
ARMS – Broilers – 2011	Operations that produced broilers for meat and had at least 1,000 broilers onsite at any time during the year	95% of broiler production[3]	2011 ARMS included 15,468 growers compared with 16,046 in 2007[4]	AL, AR, CA, DE, GA,KY, LA, MD, MS, MO, NC, OK, PA, SC, TN, TX, VA

[1] Ending-year all-hog inventory reported in the Agricultural Resource Management Survey (ARMS) as a percent of the December 1 all-hog inventory reported by USDA, National Agricultural Statistics Service (NASS) (Hogs and Pigs, 2004 and 2009). The NASS target population consists of operations with one or more hogs onsite at any time during the year.

[2] Hog operations reported in the ARMS as a percent of hog operations reported by NASS (Farms, Land in Farms, and Livestock Operations, 2005 and 2010).

[3] Annual broiler production in the ARMS (MacDonald, 2008) as a percent of broiler production reported by NASS, 2007 and 2012.

[4] The number of broiler operations is only reported by NASS in the Census of Agriculture.

Source: USDA, Economic Research Service, Agricultural Resource Management Survey data.

Only the broiler and hog ARMS commodities surveys in the years shown in Table 2 include questions specifically about antibiotic use. The hog surveys ask whether the operator provided antibiotics in feed or water for growth promotion, disease prevention, and/or disease treatment. These questions are asked regarding breeding, nursery, and finishing hogs. Due to production contracts common in the industry, hog farm operators may receive feed from integrators. Therefore, the operators may not know the content of the feed, including whether antibiotics are present. In the 2009 hog survey, operators have the option of stating they do not know if antibiotics are provided "in feed or water." In the 2004 hog survey, operators are not given the option of stating they do not know, but can leave the question blank.

The ARMS broiler surveys ask a single question about whether the broilers were raised without antibiotics in their "feed or water," excluding antibiotics administered due to illness. It is not possible to distinguish from the survey whether operators administered antibiotics for purposes of disease prevention or growth promotion. Production contracts dominate the broiler industry, and many farm operators may not know if the feed provided by contractors contains antibiotics. In the survey years used in this report, operators are given the option to state that they do not know if the feed or water contains antibiotics used for purposes other than disease treatment.

The ARMS does not distinguish between traditional antibiotics and ionophores, which are not used in human medicine (see Box, Definitions of "Production-Purpose Uses" and "Antibiotic," p. 2).

National Animal Health Monitoring Survey (NAHMS)

The USDA's Animal and Plant Health Inspection Service (APHIS) conducts the NAHMS in conjunction with NASS. The NAHMS shares several features with the ARMS. The NAHMS is also nationally representative, and in each year the NAHMS focuses on a different portion of the livestock industry. Table 3 shows the years, commodities, and basic characteristics of the NAHMS reports accessed in this study.

The NAHMS differs from the ARMS largely in purpose. The NAHMS surveys focus on animal health and management, including morbidity and mortality, disease occurrence, and disease prevention practices. The NAHMS surveys collect more detailed information on specific antibiotics used in production, including by specific purpose. The information collected on antibiotics varies greatly across commodities and across time for the same commodities. Several surveys record, for example, whether or not antibiotics were administered via feed, water, or injection and the purpose of their administration. Some of the NAHMS documents also report statistics on the specific type of antibiotic used.

The NAHMS and ARMS also differ somewhat in sample design. The ARMS focuses on hog production operations with 25 or more head versus the NAHMS focus on operations with 100 or more head. Thus, the ARMS contains smaller operations on average than NAHMS. This may influence comparison of statistics from the two surveys if characteristics of smaller operations differ from those of larger operations.

INDUSTRY STRUCTURE AND ANTIBIOTIC USE

How growth-promoting antibiotics are used, who makes the decision to use them, how restrictions on production-purpose uses of antibiotics would be felt in the industry, and how policies would be implemented depend on the structure and organization of livestock production. While antibiotic use and industry structure are related in a complex manner, we focus on possible effects of restrictions on production-purpose antibiotics on livestock operations characterized by three common organizational features:

- ***Vertical integration*** matters in terms of who bears the cost of production-purpose antibiotic restrictions and how a policy will be implemented. Vertical integration occurs when large firms or single entities control all or several parts of meat production, from feed mills to the retail level. Integrators contract with growers and dictate feed formulations, including administration of growth-promoting antibiotics. Integrators bear the cost of feed, veterinary services, and medication; restrictions on antibiotic use that change any of these inputs will entail changes in costs for integrators. Integrators may also dictate other aspects of production, such as housing specifics or production practices, but growers are responsible for the cost of these inputs, which may also be affected by restrictions in antibiotic use. The level of integration has a bearing on the relative ease with which policies can be implemented. Integrators in certain industries each control a large portion of production; fewer decision makers influencing larger shares of production can institute changes more easily than thousands of entities covering small shares of production. Vertical integration is nearly universal in the broiler sector, is increasingly common in the hog sector, has some influence in the beef sector, and is not common in dairy.

Table 3. Characteristics of National Animal Health Monitoring System (NAHMS) reports used

Report	Targeted population	States included	Percentage of U.S. inventory represented by included States	Percentage of U.S. operations represented by included States
NAHMS – Swine – 2006 – Parts II and III: Reference of Swine Health and Health Management Practices in the United States	Operations with 100 or more pigs	AR, CO,IL, IN, IA, KS, MI, MN, MO, NE, NC, OH, OK, PA, SD, TX, WI	94.2% of inventory on operations with 100 or more pigs	93.6% of operations with 100 or more pigs
NAHMS – Beef 2007-08 – Antimicrobial Drug Use and Antimicrobial Resistance on U.S. Cow-calf Operations	Operations with beef cows	AL, AR, CA, CO, FL, GA, ID, IA, KS, KY, LA, MS, MO, MT, NE, NM, ND, OK, OR, SD, TN, TX, VA, WY	79.6% of operations with beef-cows	87.8% of beef-cow inventory
NAHMS – Feedlots 2011 – Part I: Management Practices on U.S. Feedlots with a Capacity of 1,000 or More Head	Operations with a capacity of 1,000 or more head	AZ, CA, CO, ID, IA, KS, NE, NM, OK, SD, TX, WA	Over 95% of inventory in large feedlots	Not reported

NAHMS – Feedlots 2011 – Part II: Management Practices on U.S. Feedlots with a Capacity of Fewer than 1,000 Head	Operations with a capacity of fewer than 1,000 head	IL, IN, IA, KS, MI, MN, MO, NE, OH, PA, SD, TX, WI	Selected States covered 85.4% of feedlots with fewer than 500 head*	Selected States covered 90.5% of cattle in inventory on feedlots with fewer than 500 head*
NAHMS – Dairy 2007—Parts I and III: Reference of Dairy Cattle Health and Management Practices in the United States	All operations with at least one milk cow	CA, ID, IN, IA, KY, MI, MN, MO, NM, NY, OH, PA, TX, VA, VT, WA, WI	82% of milk cow inventory	79.3% of operations with milk cows
NAHMS – Dairy Heifer Raiser 2011	No initial list of all heifer-raising operations from which to sample	CA, CO, ID, IA, IN, KS, KY, MI, MN, MO, NM, NY, ND, OH, PA, TX, VA, VT, WA, WI	Not reported	Not reported

* See USDA, APHIS, 2013b, p. 56, for explanation of why feedlots with fewer than 500 head were used as a sample frame instead of feedlots with fewer than 1,000 head.

Source: Compiled by USDA, Economic Research Service from NAHMS data.

- ***Production organized around the lifecycles of the animals*** –In this arrangement, which specializes in different phases of production and antibiotic use varying across the stages of animal growth, restrictions may have heterogeneous effects on different types of operations and may disrupt supply chains (at least in the short term).
- ***Geographic concentration of the industry,*** as well as the specific location, has a bearing on which areas of the country would be most impacted by policy-induced changes. Spatial concentration also impacts the implementation of the FDA policy to require a veterinarian's prescription for all medically important antibiotics; geographically dispersed, independent producers may have more trouble obtaining veterinary services than highly concentrated, vertically integrated ones. Livestock veterinarians may only operate in specific areas and may be unwilling or unable to travel to some operations.

Hogs

How Is the U.S. Hog Industry Structured?

U.S. hog production has changed substantially over the last few decades, with increases in operation size, specialization, reliance on purchased feed, and use of production contracts. Between 1992 and 2009, the number of hog operations fell by over two-thirds, from over 240,000 to about 71,000, while the U.S. hog inventory has remained relatively stable (McBride and Key, 2013). Large operations account for an increasing share of total output. From 1992 to 2009, the share of the hog and pig inventory on farms with 2,000 head or more increased from less than 30 percent to 86 percent.

Hog production can be divided into four phases (Figure 3): (1) breeding sows and maintaining them during gestation; (2) farrowing, the process of birth to weaning; (3) the nursery phase, which includes the care of pigs immediately after weaning until about 30-80 pounds; and (4) finishing, which includes feeding pigs from 30-80 pounds to a slaughter weight of 225-300 pounds. Hog operations are classified according to the phase of the animal's life in which they specialize. "Farrow-to-finish" operations cover all phases. "Farrow-to-feeder" operations cover phases 1 through 3. "Feeder-to-finish" or "finish only" operations cover just phase 4. "Weanling-to-feeder" operations covers just phase 3, while "farrow-to-weaning" operations cover phases 1 and 2.

While most hog production once occurred on farrow-to-finish operations that raised animals from birth to market, many operations now specialize in specific phases of production (Table 4). In 2009, only 24 percent of hog operations were considered "farrow-to-finish." In addition to greater specialization in separate lifecycle phases, individual hog operations are becoming less diversified in terms of commodities produced, with an increasing share of the farm's value of production coming from the hog enterprise. For operations with hogs, the share of farm product value from hogs increased from 46 percent in 1992 to 70 percent in 2009. Over the same period, the percent of farm-grown grain fed to hogs fell from 49 percent to 26 percent (McBride and Key, 2013).

A majority of hog production occurs in the Heartland States, particularly Iowa (Table 4), but there is some geographic variation with respect to the stages. Farrow-to-finish and feeder-to-finish operations are more often located in the Heartland, coinciding with abundant supplies of corn and soybeans for feed. While wean-to-feeder operations specializing in nursery pigs were also

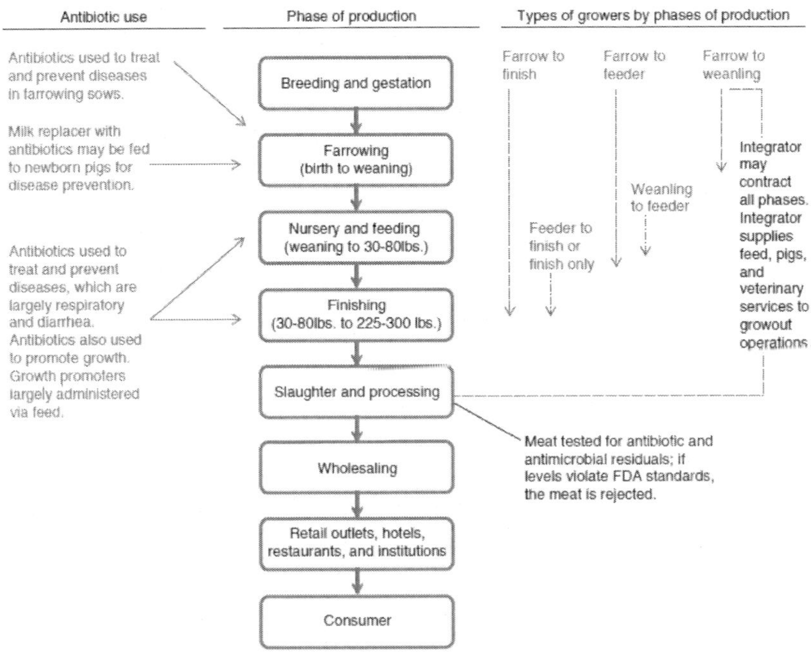

Source: USDA, Economic Research Service.

Figure 3. Phases of pork production and antibiotic use.

concentrated in the Heartland, nearly a quarter of such operations were in the Southern Seaboard. Farrow-to-feeder operations were most prominent in the Western regions. Younger pigs in both types of operations are often transferred to the Heartland for finishing (McBride and Key, 2013). Most slaughter occurs in the regions with the most production, particularly of finishing hogs; in 2012, slightly more than half (52 percent) of hog slaughter occurred in the four Heartland States of Iowa, Illinois, Indiana, and Missouri (USDA, NASS, 2012a).

Increases in scale and specialization have coincided with a rising use of production contracts and vertical integration. A production contract is an arrangement between the pig owner (contractor) and the farmer who cares for the animals. Operations with production contracts accounted for only 5 percent of hog production in 1992, but 71 percent of production in 2009 (McBride and Key, 2013). Nearly 80 percent of production on feeder-to-finish farms was under production contracts in 2009.

Contractors include packers (slaughter and processing companies) and "integrators"–individuals who contract with a number of growers and also have marketing arrangements for the hogs with packers. Some contractors operate on a very large scale. The 5 largest hog integrators account for about a third of production, and the 20 next largest handle 22 percent, leaving 45 percent to be handled by several thousand small integrators and independent producers (statistics generated from Freese, 2013, and USDA, NASS, 2014a).

Table 4. Characteristics of hog production, by producer type, 2009

	Type of hog producer					
	All	**Farrow to finish**	**Farrow to feeder**	**Feeder to finish**	**Farrow to wean**	**Wean to feeder**
Percent of operations	100	24	5	47	4	7
Percentage of operations using production contracts	48	2	9	74	46	98
Farm production from hog sales or removals ($1,000) (average by farm)	938	609	208	1,260	1,040	832
Percentage of farm production from hogs sales or contract removals (average by farm)	70	58	78	71	84	76
Region						
Heartland	62	56	12	76	50	60
Northern Crescent	11	16	22	9	7	7
Eastern Uplands	4	4	15	1	26	6
Southern Seaboard	10	5	8	9	7	23
Western region	13	19	42	5	10	4

Source: Key and McBride, 2013. See Key and McBride for a map denoting regions. Generally, for this data, the Heartland refers to the Midwestern States including Iowa, Illinois, Indiana, and parts of Ohio, Missouri, and other States. The Northern Crescent refers to portions of States adjacent to the Great Lakes. The Eastern Uplands refers to portions of the Appalachian Mountain States, including parts of Tennessee and Kentucky. The Eastern Uplands also includes portions of Arkansas, eastern Oklahoma, and southern Missouri. The Southern Seaboard extends from Virginia to portions of Alabama, excluding Florida and some seaboard portions of Georgia and South Carolina. The Western region includes portions of Texas, Utah, Colorado, South Dakota, Nebraska, and Kansas.

With most hogs raised under production contracts, antibiotic use decisions are primarily made by a limited number of integrators, not contract growers, and integrators will also bear the immediate impact of costs associated with any changes in feed formulation or consumption following restrictions on use of antibiotics for production purposes. Compliance efforts will therefore focus on integrators, and integrators' immediate efforts to comply are likely to focus on elements under their direct control, such as feed formulation and breeding. Changes in grower investments in capital or equipment, or in on-farm practices carried out by growers, are likely to require adjustments to contracts.

How Are Antibiotics Used in the Nursery Stage of Hog Production?

The uses of antibiotics in disease control, prevention, and treatment and in growth promotion differ over the swine lifecycle. In the farrowing phase, sows may be treated with antibiotics to prevent or treat infections associated with difficult births. At 1 to 3 days of age, piglets may be given antibiotics to manage bacterial problems near the umbilical cord and in joints (*National Hog Farmer*, 2011). Bacteria-induced diarrhea in piglets is a particular problem in nursery facilities. In 2006, 13.2 percent of preweaning deaths were caused by scours (another name for diarrhea), making it the leading disease cause of death for preweaned piglets.[4] Antibiotic therapies are frequently used to treat diarrhea in the preweaning stage. In the nursery and finishing stages, respiratory problems are the most prevalent disease-induced causes of death (53.7 and 60.1 percent, respectively). Antibiotics are frequently injected to treat respiratory problems in these stages (USDA APHIS, 2007b and 2007c).

Despite the fact that antibiotics for growth promotion have a larger impact in nursery pigs than in finishing hogs (Dritz et al., 2002), use of growth-promoting antibiotics in the nursery stage is far from universal. The NAHMS data indicate that for growth promotion in 2006, 24.5 percent of sites with nursery-age hogs administered antibiotics in feed, 0.5 percent in water, and 1.4 percent via injection (Table 5).[5] In 2006, a larger portion of operations administered antibiotics to nursery-age hogs for disease prevention than for growth promotion: 50.9 percent of sites via feed, 14.6 percent via water, and 20.9 percent via injection. The percentage of sites feeding nursery-age pigs antibiotics for growth promotion appears to be declining according to prior NAHMS data; in 2000, 82 percent of sites with nursery-age pigs administered antibiotics in feed for growth promotion (USDA, APHIS, 2002, p. 42), compared to 24.5 percent in 2006.

Table 5. Percentage of sites that gave any pigs an antimicrobial or feed additive, by type of pig, primary reason given, and route of administration, 2006

	Percentage of sites with:					
	Nursery-age pigs			Grower/finisher		
	Route of administration			Route of administration		
	Injection	Feed	Water	Injection	Feed	Water
Growth promotion	1.4	24.5	0.5	1.0	55.1	0.2
Disease prevention	20.9	50.9	14.6	10.8	37.5	3.7
Respiratory disease treatment	48.6	17.0	17.7	63.7	29.0	42.4
Enteric disease treatment	19.1	14.8	9.9	15.9	17.1	15.8
Polyserositis/meningitis treatment	25.1	0.7	4.8	14.3	0.0	0.9
Parasite treatment	0.0	6.8	0.4	0.0	0.0	0.0
Other treatment	10.4	0.1	0.7	12.1	1.6	0.6
Any reason	83.1	82.3	40.3	75.6	83.6	47.9

Note: The statistics indicate the percentage of the sites using the treatment, not the percentage of pigs treated at the facility. Source: USDA, Animal and Plant Health Inspection Service (APHIS). 2007b; National Animal Health Monitoring System (NAHMS), Swine 2006 - Part II: Reference of Swine Health and Health Management Practices in the United States, 2006, pp. 46, 48, 51, 58, 61, and 64.

The 2009 ARMS data also reflect the fact that a sizable percentage of nursery-hog operations do not use antibiotics for growth promotion. Table 6 reports the percentage of operations with 25 or more hogs that administered antibiotics via feed or water to hogs at different stages of growth. Among operations with nursery pigs, 33 percent reported administering antibiotics to nursery pigs for growth promotion, 62 percent for disease prevention, and 48 percent for disease treatment purposes. Assuming that these operations administered antibiotics to all hogs, this constitutes 23, 9, and 59 percent of nursery hogs sold or removed.[6] However, between 5 and 8 percent of operations reported that they did not know whether antibiotics were administered via feed or water for the stated purpose; their operations handled between 17 and 26 percent of nursery hogs removed or sold. Overall, these 2009 ARMS data suggest that between 23 and 49 percent of nursery hogs sold or removed received antibiotics for growth promotion.

The percentages of farms with nursery-age hogs who were feeding antibiotics for different purposes vary somewhat between the 2006 NAHMS data and the 2009 ARMS data (tables 5 and 6). The 2006 NAHMS reports that 24.5 percent of operations with nursery hogs administered antibiotics in feed for growth promotion, while the 2009 ARMS reports the percentage administered antibiotics in feed or water for growth promotion at between 33 and 41 percent. Both studies suggest that the majority of sites with nursery hogs do not use antibiotics in feed for growth promotion. The difference in NAHMS and ARMS percentages might arise from differences in the survey years, such as in sample-weighting protocols, methods of gathering information, specific question asked, and the composition of the sample.[7]

Table 6. Proportion of hog producers using antibiotics, by type of hog and purpose of use, 2009

	Percentage of operations that use antibiotics for:				
Type of hog	Growth promotion	Disease prevention	Either growth promotion or disease prevention	Disease treatment	Any use
Nursery hogs					
Operations					
Yes	33	62	65	48	73
Don't know	8	5	5	5	5
Head sold or removed					
Yes	23	59	60	59	77
Don't know	26	20	21	18	17
Finishing hogs					
Operations					
Yes	30	44	50	44	61
Don't know	16	14	14	13	12
Head sold or removed					
Yes	40	51	59	61	74
Don't know	22	20	20	18	17

Notes: The "yes" responses in the "Either…" and the "Any use" categories are the sum of the responses of "yes" to use for at least one indicated purpose. The "no" responses are those who respond "no" to use for any of the indicated purposes. The "don't know" responses are those who respond "don't know" to use for all of the indicated purposes or respond "no" or "don't know" in combination.

Source: ERS calculations from Agricultural Resource Management Survey (ARMS) Hogs 2009 data.

Table 7. Proportion of hogs sold or removed from operations reporting antibiotic use, by reason for use, contract status, and type of hog; 2009

	Administration of antibiotics via feed or water					
	Yes		Don't know		No	
	Contract	Non-Contract	Contract	Non-Contract	Contract	Non-Contract
Nursery hogs sold or removed						
Growth promotion	0.22	0.28	0.29	0.07	0.48	0.65
Disease prevention	0.55	0.86	0.22	0.05	0.22	0.10
Disease treatment	0.55	0.86	0.20	0.05	0.22	0.10
Finishing hogs sold or removed						
Growth promotion	0.32	0.57	0.30	0.05	0.38	0.38
Disease prevention	0.45	0.65	0.27	0.05	0.28	0.30
Disease treatment	0.58	0.67	0.24	0.05	0.18	0.28

Source: ERS calculations from Agricultural Resource Management Survey (ARMS) 2009 Hogs. For example, 22 percent of nursery hogs sold or removed from operations with production contracts reported to have received antibiotics for growth promotion.

Reporting of antibiotic use varies by whether there is a production contract. In 2009, 83 percent of nursery hogs and 64 percent of finishing hogs were removed under contract. The proportion of both nursery and finishing hogs reportedly being administered antibiotics via feed or water for growth promotion, disease prevention, or disease treatment is lower for contract than noncontract production (Table 7). However, the proportion of hogs removed from operations stating they do not know whether antibiotics are administered is much higher for contract production. This makes it difficult to ascertain whether contract production is more or less likely to involve the use of antibiotics.

While ARMS surveys of the U.S. hog industry in 2004 and 2009 allow for comparisons across time, discerning trends is difficult due to changes in the proportion of operations not reporting whether or not they used antibiotics or those declaring they do not know if antibiotics were used (Figure 4).[8] Among producers with nursery-age pigs, the percentages of nursery hogs reportedly administered antibiotics for growth promotion, disease prevention, and disease treatment all fell slightly. However, the portions of nursery hogs falling in the grouped "don't know or missing" category rose approximately fourfold for each of these uses. Hence, it is difficult to assess whether there were any changes in use from the ARMS data.[9]

How Are Antibiotics Used in the Finishing Stage of Hog Production?

Some illnesses are more common in older hogs than nursery pigs. In the grower/finisher stage, respiratory infections are the largest cause of death among hogs (USDA, APHIS, 2007); reflecting this, 63.7 percent of hog-finishing sites injected antibiotics for respiratory disease treatment in 2006 (Table 5).

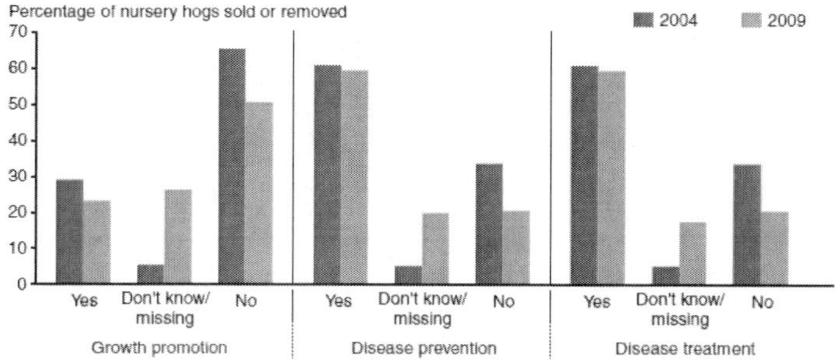

Source: USDA, Economic Research Service from Agricultural Resource Management Survey (ARMS) data, Hogs 2004 and 2009 data.

Figure 4. Percentage of nursery-age hogs sold or removed from operations that administered antibiotics via feed or water, by purpose, 2004 and 2009.

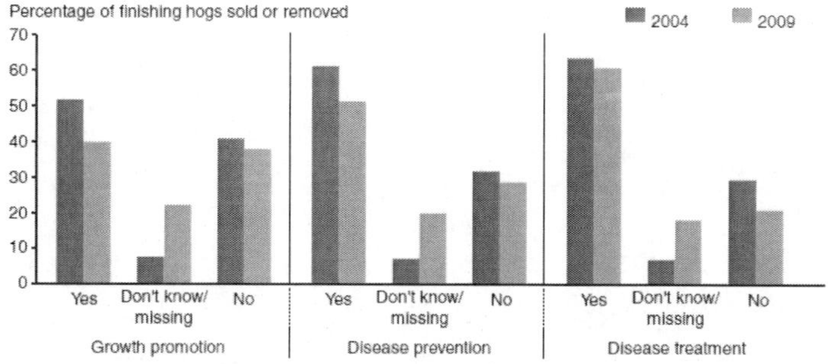

Source: USDA, Economic Research Service from Agricultural Resource Management Survey (ARMS) data, Hogs 2004 and 2009 data.

Figure 5. Percentage of finishing hogs sold or removed from operations that administered antibiotics via feed or water, by purpose, 2004 and 2009.

The percentage of finishing hog operations using growth-promoting antibiotics is approximately half and has declined since 2000. The NAHMS data suggest that 55.1 percent of sites with grower/finisher hogs administered antibiotics via feed for growth promotion in 2006, while 0.2 percent did so via water and 1.0 percent via injection (Table 5). The percentage of operations feeding antibiotics for growth promotion was lower than in 2000, when it was 63.7 percent (USDA, APHIS, 2002, p. 51).

According to 2009 ARMS data (Table 6), 30 percent of producers with finishing hogs reported using antibiotics for growth promotion. This constituted 40 percent of finishing hogs, assuming all hogs raised by these producers were given antibiotics for this purpose. However, 16 percent of operations (with 22 percent of hogs) also reported that they did not know if antibiotics were administered for growth promotion. The percentage of operations administering antibiotics for disease prevention was 44 percent, constituting 51 percent of hogs. For disease treatment, these numbers are 44 percent of operations administering antibiotics (for 61 percent of hogs). Note that due to the large percentages of respondents supplying "don't know" answers, the percentages of hogs fed antibiotics for growth promotion could be between 40 and 66 percent.

Again, there are discrepancies in antibiotic use rates between the ARMS and NAHMS data sources. For example, the 2006 NAHMS data shows that 55.1 percent of finisher operations administered antibiotics in feed (and 0.2 percent in water) for growth promotion (Table 5), compared with between 30 and 46 percent in feed or water according to the 2009 ARMS data (Table 6).[10] The statistics from both surveys suggest that use of growth-promoting antibiotics is not universal in the finishing hog sector but may be higher than for nursery hogs.

For operations with finishing hogs, the ARMS data show decreases between 2004 and 2009 in the proportion of hogs reportedly supplied antibiotics for growth promotion, disease prevention, and disease treatment (52 to 40 percent, 61 to 51 percent, and 64 to 61 percent, respectively) (Figure 5). Again, note that the proportion of "don't know" or missing responses increased about threefold over the period, making statements about trends based on ARMS data difficult.

Production Practices by Antibiotic Use in Hog Production

There appears to be a positive correlation between production practices that affect animal hygiene and the use of antibiotics for growth promotion. ARMS data from 2009 show that hog producers using antibiotics for growth promotion are more likely to employ a set of hygiene-promoting practices. For example, nursery hog producers who use antibiotics for growth promotion are more likely to use all-in, all-out systems—starting a group of hogs in a nursery facility at the same time and then removing them together—and are also more likely to engage in production practices aimed at disease prevention (Table 8). All-in, all-out systems can help reduce the spread of disease. Antibiotic users are also more likely to employ other hygiene-related measures, such as securing Pork Quality Assurance Plus certification, using rodent control around facilities, cleaning transportation vehicles before loading hogs, and "bird-proofing" production facilities with screening.

A similar pattern emerges for operations with finishing hogs: for both farrow-to-finish and feeder-to-finish operations, facilities that administer antibiotics for growth promotion are more likely to employ hygiene-related practices such as all-in, all-out systems in their growout facilities, to have Pork Quality Assurance Plus certification, and to use rodent control (Table 9). Antibiotic users are also more likely to use split-sex (feeding male and female pigs separately) and phase feeding (adapting feed ingredients to changing nutrient requirements).

A higher risk of disease may be leading farms to adopt antibiotics for growth promotion along with hygiene practices. Operations facing a lower disease threat may not need to adopt either measure.

Broilers

How Is the U.S. Broiler Industry Structured?

Broilers young chickens bred and fed for meat—account for two-thirds of poultry-sector cash receipts; turkeys and eggs account for most of the rest. In 2012, there were 42,226 operations with broilers in their inventory; 89 percent of the 8.5 billion broilers produced came from the 33 percent of operations selling at least 300,000 head (USDA, NASS, 2014b). Most broiler production occurs in the Southeastern States. Almost all U.S. broiler production is carried out through production contracts between growers and integrators. Twenty integrators, who combine feed mills, hatcheries, and processing plants with contract-grower operations, accounted for 96 percent of all broilers produced in the United States in 2011. Unlike in the hog industry, there are virtually no independent producers in broiler production and very few small integrators (MacDonald, 2014). Compliance with regulations will therefore be focused on integrators.

Table 8. Production practices of operations with nursery hogs, by use of antibiotics as a growth promotant in nursery hogs, 2009

	Percent of all operations with nursery hogs		Percent of farrow-to-wean operations	
	Use of antibiotics as growth promotant		Use of antibiotics as growth promotant	
Production practice	Yes	No	Yes	No
All-in, all-out system used in farrowing facilities	32	32	72	47
All-in, all-out system used in nursery facilities	72	52***	72	29
Pork Quality Assurance Plus certification	83	58***	46	77
Cats or wildlife have access to production facilities or feed- preparation areas	45	50	0	36
Routine rodent control program in and around hog production facilities	92	77***	94	85
Written biosecurity plan	25	27	21	46
Vehicles used to transport hogs cleaned and disin-fected before loading hogs	66	53***	100	79
Production facilities "bird-proofed" with screening	59	46**	100	68

*Denotes that means are statistically different at the 90% level. **Denotes statistical significance at the 95% level.

***Denotes statistical significance at the 99% level.

Source: ERS calculations using Agricultural Resource Management Survey (ARMS) 2009 data.

Like hog production, broiler production is divided into phases corresponding to the lifecycle of the chicken (Figure 6). Integrators provide contract growers with chicks, feed, and veterinary services and collect broilers for delivery to their processing plants. The chicks are delivered to growers from hatcheries that are owned by the integrators. In turn, the hatcheries receive eggs from contract "breeder-broiler" farms. Integrators also own or contract with primary breeder companies for breeding stock.

Table 9. Production practices of operations with finishing hogs, by use of antibiotics as a growth promotant in finishing hogs, 2009

	Percent of farrow-to-finish operations		Percent of feeder-to-finish operations	
	Use of antibiotics as growth promotant		Use of antibiotics as growth promotant	
Production practice	Yes	No	Yes	No
All-in, all-out system in growout facilities	51	30**	88	78***
Split-sex feeding	20	7**	31	20**
Phase feeding	75	38***	91	71***
Pork Quality Assurance Plus certification	86	52***	88	73***
Cats or wildlife have access to production facilities or feed preparation areas	66	70	20	23
Routine rodent control program in and around hog production facilities	88	71**	95	82***
Written biosecurity plan	26	12**	47	48
Vehicles used to transport hogs cleaned and disin-fected before loading hogs	41	36	81	81
Production facilities "bird-proofed" with screening	50	20***	82	78
Growing-finishing hogs dewormed	76	80	36	38

*Denotes that means are statistically different at the 90% level. **Denotes statistical significance at the 95% level.

***Denotes statistical significance at the 99% level.

Source: ERS calculations from Agricultural Resource Management Survey (ARMS) 2009 data.

Contract growers tend to be relatively small and specialized family farms, with average sales (gross cash income) of $232,000 in 2011, 70 percent of which comes from fees for broiler production. The average size of an individual grower operation has steadily increased, with the average number of birds removed in a year reaching 504,180 in 2011.

Integrator-owned trucks transport feed and chicks to grow out and broiler-breeder farms, eggs to hatcheries, live birds to processing plants, and chicken products to further-processing plants. Because of the expense of truck transportation, farms, mills, hatcheries, and plants must locate in a network within close proximity to one another—in 2011, 90 percent of all broilers were raised within 60 miles of the processing plant (MacDonald, 2014).

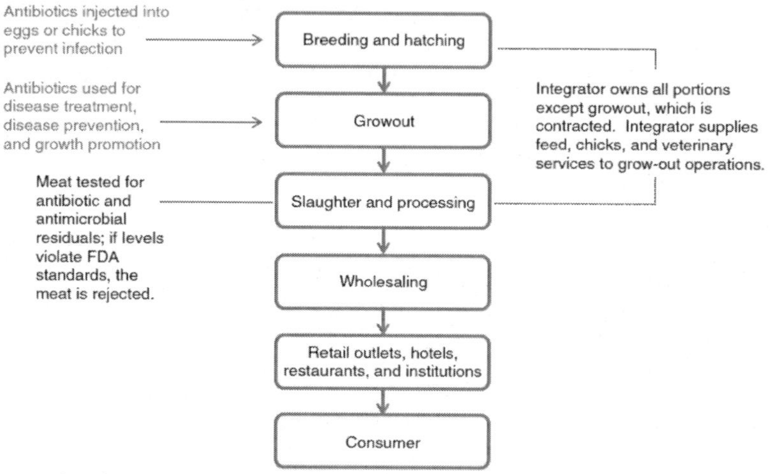

Source: USDA, Economic Research Service.

Figure 6. Phases of broiler production and antibiotic use.

Integrators provide growers with feed and veterinary services and decide whether and how to administer antibiotics on the farms. Because integrators make decisions about feed formulations, they will bear the immediate costs of restrictions on antibiotics used in feed. Integrators also manage breeding programs and therefore make the major decisions regarding flock genetics. Integrators specify and enforce production practices to be carried out on farms and set specifications for acceptable house designs. Contract growers provide labor, management, and housing services, and the growers ultimately make the final decisions for investments in housing designs and equipment (although often with incentives from integrators). Growers are responsible for increased costs associated with these changes; any cost increases will likely lead to adjustments in contracts.

How Are Antibiotics Used in Broiler Production?

Salmonella, E. coli, and Clostridium are major disease concerns among poultry growers. Antibiotics may be used to treat sick birds, and flocks may also be given a course of antibiotics in feed or water to prevent the spread of disease when outbreaks have been detected in nearby houses or farms.

Antibiotics are injected into eggs or chicks to improve early viability and are regularly fed to poultry to treat diseases, prevent infections, and promote growth (NRC, 1999).

In the ARMS broiler surveys in 2006 and 2011, producers were asked whether they raised their broilers *without* antibiotics in their feed or water unless the birds were sick. This would include both purposes of growth promotion and disease prevention. In 2011, nearly half of contract growout operations (48 percent) reported that broilers were only given antibiotics when they were sick. Those operations also accounted for 48 percent of birds and associated liveweight production under contract, which implies that larger contract growers were no more likely to provide antibiotics for growth promotion or disease prevention than smaller contract operations. This large share cannot be attributed to organic production, which forgoes the use of antibiotics but constitutes only 2 percent of production (MacDonald, 2014). Approximately a third (32 percent) of operators state that they do not know if they provided antibiotics via feed or water for purposes other than disease treatment. Hence, the proportion of operations that report that they only supplied antibiotics for disease treatment could be as high as 80 percent. These statistics suggest that in 2011 between 20 and 52 percent of operations used antibiotics for nontherapeutic reasons.

Comparing the 2006 and 2011 ARMS data shows that the percentage of broiler producers who raised birds *without* antibiotics (except in the event of illness in the flock) rose from 42 percent in 2006 to 48 percent in 2011 (Figure 7). Percentages are similar for farms, number of birds, or the pounds of production (by liveweight). Note that in each year about a third of producers report that they "don't know" if antibiotics were provided in feed or water (except for disease treatment). As discussed, this may be because integrators supply feed, and thus producers may be unaware of the feed formulation. Because the survey consistently allows producers to report they "don't know" about use and the percentage of operations reporting that they "don't know" remains fairly constant, we can have some confidence in the trends in usage rates compared to the trends in the ARMS data for hogs.

These declines in antibiotic use in broilers are consistent with evidence indicating a long-term shift away from use of antibiotics for growth promotion in broiler production. Chapman and Johnson (2002) used data on feed formulations provided to growers and found that 33 percent did not include antibiotics in 2000, compared with 2 percent in 1995. As noted earlier, a number of major retailers have begun requiring that their suppliers provide

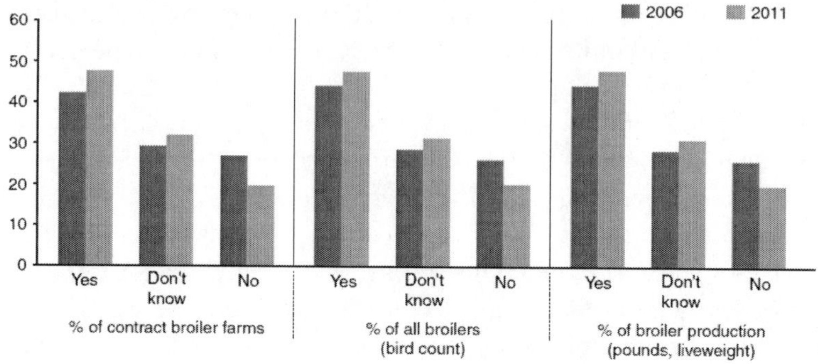

Source: Agricultural Resource Management Survey (ARMS) broiler survey data, 2006, 2011. ARMS asked respondents if they used antibiotics only in the event of illness, the question to which the "Yes" responders were replying. "Birds" refers to broiler headcount; "production" refers to total live weight of broilers.

Figure 7. Birds raised by U.S. contract broiler producers without antibiotics in food or water (except in cases of illness), 2006 and 2011.

products raised without antibiotics for growth promotion. In addition, more supermarket chains have been offering products labeled as "antibiotic-free" or "raised without antibiotics."

Production Practices by Antibiotic Use in Broiler Production

In broiler production, a range of investments and practices can be used to reduce the incidence of on-farm diseases. Broiler producers who only use antibiotics for disease treatment appear somewhat more likely to use production practices that could improve animal hygiene, although responses of "don't know" hinder drawing definitive conclusions (Table 10). Growers who indicated they did not use antibiotics for growth promotion or disease prevention were more likely to treat water to control salmonella, to test their flocks for pathogens, to clean and disinfect their vehicles, and to treat litter to reduce ammonia emissions. Some growers may not be aware of practices carried out by integrators and report on the survey that they "don't know" whether the production practice is used. For example, ARMS data from 2011 show that over 50 percent of respondents did not know whether there were animal byproducts in the feed, whether their flock was tested for campylobacter, or whether their breeding flocks were vaccinated for salmonella.

Almost all broiler producers followed a rodent-control program. Similarly, nearly all producers used an all-in, all-out system, in which all chicks placed on the operation at the same time and all grown broilers removed and taken to slaughter at the same time. All-in, all-out production can make it easier to control the spread of disease since it reduces the chances of infections spreading from flock to flock. Those chances can be further reduced by cleaning and disinfecting houses between placements of flocks; in 2011, 21 percent of contract growers cleaned out and disinfected their houses after every flock removal (MacDonald, 2014).

Beef

How Is the U.S. Beef Industry Structured?

Beef cattle production is divided into three stages of production (first three boxes in Figure 8). Operations may specialize in one or more of these stages of production. The first stage is cow-calf operations, where calves are birthed and raised until weaning (around 6-9 months).[11] The second stage takes place on stocker or backgrounding operations, where weaned calves consume mostly forage for 3 to 8 months to gain 200-400 pounds. The third stage is the finishing or feedlot period, where steers and heifers are fed a combination of forage and grain to a slaughter weight of 1,000-1,500 pounds. After being fed to market weight, cattle are sent to beef processors who market beef and other products (including hides and offal). Cattle are often shipped long distances between phases of production.

The beef industry is less vertically integrated than the pork and broiler industries, due to large numbers of small-scale producers and cattle's longer production cycle. In 2012, there were 727,906 farms with 1 or more beef cows; of these, 82 percent had fewer than 50 cows and accounted for 30 percent of the 28.96 million beef cows in the United States. Larger farms were fewer in number; of farms with beef cows, 0.2 percent had 1,000 or more cows, accounting for 8 percent of cows (USDA, NASS, 2014b).

Ownership of cattle generally changes over the animals' lifecycles. In 2007, about half (49.8 percent) of cow-calf operations sold all of their calves at weaning (USDA, APHIS, 2010). Another 30 percent of cow-calf operations retained calves from 1 to 61 days past weaning, but not generally long enough for a stockering phase. Twenty percent retained ownership for over 61 days,

Table 10. Antibiotic use, production outcomes, and production practices in broiler growout facilities

Operation only used antibiotics for disease treatment			
	No	**Yes**	**Don't Know**
Number of farms	3,070	7,401	4,981
Production outcome			
Average annual production (# birds)	530,690	529,596	519,133
Flock mortality rate (%)	3.53	3.83	3.75
Feed conversion (lb. of feed per lb. of weight)	1.89	1.91	1.89
Production Practice	**% farms reporting use of production practice (% reporting "don't know" in parentheses)**		
Water treated to control salmonella after feed withdrawn	26 (5)	33 (7)	22 (12)
Use of prebiotics or probiotics in feed	21 (49)	18 (65)	7 (91)
No animal byproducts in feed	31 (51)	27 (64)	11 (84)
Test flocks for avian influenza	53 (42)	60 (36)	50 (45)
Test flocks for salmonella	46 (50)	50 (45)	29 (68)
Test flocks for campylobacter	23 (73)	25 (70)	11 (86)
Breeding flocks vaccinated for salmonella	33 (62)	36 (61)	20 (77)
Follows National Poultry Improvement Plan	48 (34)	51 (37)	47 (42)
Follows routine rodent control program	96 (1)	97 (1)	95 (1)
Follows specified animal welfare requirements	82 (11)	88 (9)	78 (2)
Uses all-in all-out production	93 (4)	96 (2)	97 (2)
Vehicles cleaned & disinfected before loading birds	30 (58)	37 (47)	26 (60)
Litter in houses windrowed and dried between flocks	31 (0)	35 (0)	28 (0)
Litter in houses treated to reduce ammonia	63 (0)	73 (0)	66 (0)
Houses cleaned and disinfected at least annually	19 (1)	21 (1)	22 (1)

Source: 2011 Agricultural Resource Management Survey, version 4. Contract growers only. For example, 18 percent of operations that only use antibiotics for disease treatment use prebiotics or probiotics in feed. Sixty-five percent of operations that only use antibiotics for disease treatment report that they "don't know" if prebiotics or probiotics are used in feed.

many of which kept the animals through a stockering phase (USDA, APHIS, 2010). Few cow-calf operations (9 percent) retained ownership of animals from birth through the feedlot stage (USDA, APHIS, 2010).

While cow-calf operations are dispersed in a vast number of farms over a wide geographic area, feedlots are more concentrated (Table 11). At one extreme, 66 feedlots with capacity greater than 50,000 head (0.10 percent of feedlots) accounted for 33 percent of fed cattle marketed in 2012. At the other extreme, 73,000 farmer-feeders with a capacity of less than 1,000 head (97 percent of feedlots) handled 11 percent of fed-cattle sales. Feedlots with at least 1,000 head constitute a small percentage of feedlots (2.8 percent) but account for the majority of cattle marketed (89 percent). Feedlots are concentrated in the Great Plains; in 2012, 71 percent of cattle on feed were sold from four States: Colorado, Kansas, Nebraska, and Texas (USDA, NASS, 2014c).

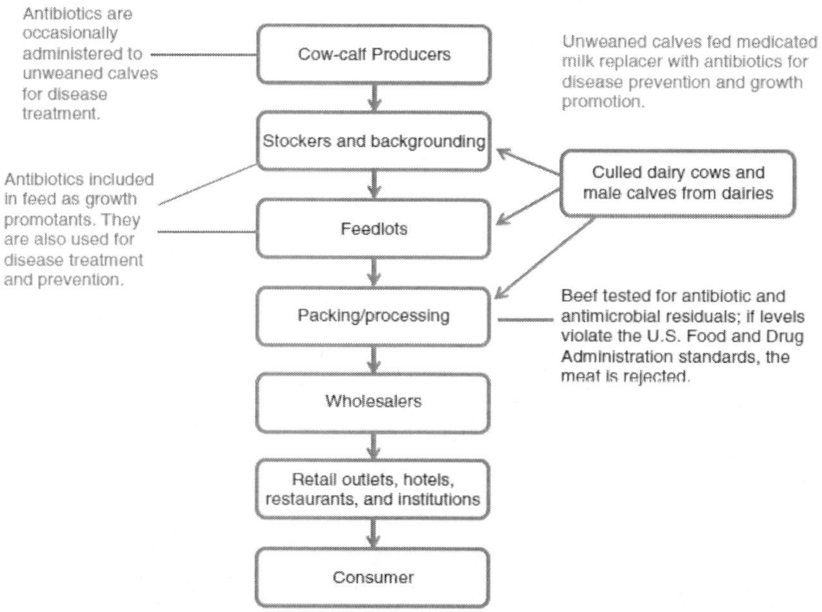

Source: USDA, Economic Research Service.

Figure 8. Beef cow life cycle and use of antibiotics in stages of production.

Table 11. Number of feedlots, inventory, and marketings by size of feedlot, 2012

	Lots(number)	Percentage of lots	Cattle marketed (1,000 head)	Percentage of cattle marketed
Less than 1,000 head	73,000	97.2%	2,854	11%
1,000 head or more	2,100	2.8%	22,028	89%
1,000-1,999	740	1.0%	678	3%
2,000-3,999	570	0.8%	1,300	5%
4,000-7,999	345	0.5%	1,800	7%
8,000-15,999	170	0.2%	2,320	9%
16,000-23,999	88	0.1%	2,150	9%
24,000-31,999	55	0.1%	1,880	8%
32,000-49,999	66	0.1%	3,750	15%
50,000 and Over	66	0.1%	8,150	33%
All feedlots	75,100	100.0%	24,882	100%

Source: USDA, National Agricultural Statistics Service (NASS), 2014c. http://usda.mannlib.cornell. edu/usda/nass/CattOnFe//2010s/2014/CattOnFe-02-21-2014.pdf.

Table 12. Percent of cattle and calves at beef feedlot operations with 1,000 or more head by origin of cattle, by region, 2011

		Region	
	All	Central	Other
Provided for custom feeding* or joint ownership with feedlot	38.5	40.7	27.8
Purchased by feedlot via auction	28.8	27.8	33.4
Purchased by feedlot via direct sale	29.6	28.2	36.5
Born on feedlot or another operation operated solely by feedlot	1.1	1.1	1.5
Obtained from other sources	2.0	2.2	0.8

Notes: *Producer-retained ownership or investor-owned. "Central" refers to Colorado, Kansas, Oklahoma, and Texas. "Other" refers to other States surveyed, including Arizona, California, Idaho, Iowa, New Mexico, South Dakota, and Washington.

Source: USDA, Animal and Plant Health Inspection Service (APHIS), 2011, p. 21, Feedlot 2011, Part I: Management Practices on U.S. Feedlots with a Capacity of 1,000 or More Head.

Virtually all cattle on feedlots are sourced from outside the feedlot, with nearly 60 percent either purchased at auction or via direct sale (Table 12). A sizeable percentage are fully or jointly owned by others and fed at the feedlot under agreement. In 2011, 38.5 percent of cattle in 1,000-head-plus feedlots were jointly owned by the feedlot and others, or were custom fed by the feedlot for other owners. This percentage is down from 73.9 percent in 1994, due in part to increasing equity requirements and volatile profit margins (USDA, APHIS 2013c). Cattle may be transported long distances to reach auction and/or the feedlot; the average distance traveled to feedlots is 339 miles (USDA, APHIS, 2013a). Some cattle entering feedlots originate from Canada and Mexico. While culled dairy cows and other cattle from dairies are sometimes fed on feedlots, they constitute only a small share of feedlot cattle.

Beef packing (inclusive of slaughtering, processing, packaging, and distribution) is even more concentrated than the feedlot stage. In 2013, four companies accounted for 85 percent of the total volume of steer and heifer slaughter and processing (USDA, GIPSA, 2014). Processing is also regionally concentrated in Colorado, Kansas, Nebraska, and Texas; in 2012, 66 percent of beef slaughter occurred in these four states (USDA, NASS, 2014c). However, only 5.5 percent of fed cattle were owned by packers in 2013. About 30 percent were acquired by packers through cash sales, and the rest were acquired through forward contracts and marketing agreements. The last two arrangements create volume and pricing commitments and frequently specify pricing incentives related to yield and quality grades; however, they do not specify production practices in the way that more specific production contracts can.

While some supply chains exist for the production of niche-market beef (for example, organic, grass-fed, or antibiotic-free), because beef cattle production is much less vertically integrated than pork or poultry, there are many more decisionmakers for feed formulations and antibiotic use. The geographic dispersion also has practical implications for the new Veterinarian Feed Directive guidelines requiring all antibiotics to be administered via veterinary prescription. If there are few veterinarians in a region to serve multiple, widely spread farmer-feeders not connected by an integrator, then requiring veterinarian oversight for medically important antibiotics for growth promotion may prove unfeasible.

How are Antibiotics Used in Beef Cattle Production?

A minority of cow-calf operations reported using antibiotics for disease prevention or production purposes. In 2007/2008, 15.8 percent of cow-calf operations reported adding antibiotics (exclusive of ionophores) to cattle feed to prevent disease and/or promote growth (APHIS, 2012). Of these operations, most reported the reason for use as disease prevention (Table 13). Only 2.6 percent of cow-calf operations included antibiotics in feed for growth promotion for replacement heifers weaned but not yet calved, and 3.4 percent of operations included antibiotics in feed for growth promotion for calves weaned but not yet shipped for feeding or being sold as breeding stock.

Table 13. Percentage of cow/calf operations that used antibiotics, by cattle class and primary purpose of use, 2007-2008

Primary purpose	Percentage of operations
Any purpose	15.8
Preweaned calves	
Prevent respiratory disease	8.0
Other	1.1
Any	8.5
Replacement heifers weaned but not yet calved	
Prevent respiratory disease	9.6
Promote growth	2.6
Other	0.3
Any	9.9
Other calves weaned but not yet shipped for feeding or sold as breeding stock	
Prevent respiratory disease	11.6
Promote growth	3.4
Other	0.3
Any	11.8

Notes: 15.8% of operations used antibiotics with or without decoquinate/ionophores in cattle feed.

Source: USDA, Animal and Plant Health Inspection Service (APHIS), 2010, Beef 2007-08 Part IV: Reference of Beef Cow- calf Management Practices in the United States, 2007-08.

Because of the stress from travel and from commingling with animals sourced from various locations, cattle arriving at feedlots may be at greater risk for illness. Upon arrival, they are often vaccinated and given antibiotics, implanted with artificial hormones, and/or treated for parasites (Table 14). In 2011, 50.4 percent of large-scale feedlots injected cattle and calves with antibiotics; this amounts to about a quarter of cattle and calves at large-scale feedlots that are being injected. Percentages are fairly similar for operations with fewer than 1,000 head. These injections treat sick cattle or serve as short-term preventive measures.

While at the feedlot, cattle subject to respiratory and digestive-tract diseases are given antibiotics to treat or prevent illness. Antimicrobials, including ionophores and coccidiostats, are also often added to feed to aid growth and improve feed efficiency.[12] In 2011, 90.5 percent of feedlots with 1,000 or more head fed the cattle an ionophore, and 44.7 percent fed them a coccidiostat (Table 15). For smaller feedlots with less than 1,000 head, these percentages were substantially lower (28.7 and 17.1 percent, respectively).

Table 14. For feedlots that initially processed cattle and calves as a group, percentage of feedlots and cattle and calves by procedures performed at initial processing, 2011

	Size of feedlot			
	1,000 or more head		Fewer than 1,000 head	
	Percent of feedlots with 1,000 or more head	Percent of cattle and calves at feedlots with 1,000 or more head	Percent of feedlots with fewer than 1,000 head	Percent of cattle and calves at feedlots with fewer than 1,000 head
Vaccinated against respiratory diseases	96.0	96.0	76.7	92.6
Vaccinated against clostridial diseases	77.3	71.6	66.4	73.4
Given an injectable antibiotic	50.4	26.0	42.0	31.0
Implanted with growth-promoting hormone	78.7	84.4	42.1	56.2
Treated for parasites	94.5	91.4	84.6	83.8

Source: USDA, Animal and Plant Health Inspection Service (APHIS), 2013a, pp. 37 and 38, Feedlot 2011 Part I: Management Practices on U.S. Feedlots with a Capacity of 1,000 or More Head. USDA, APHIS, 2013b, pp. 22 and 23, Feedlot 2011 Part II: Management Practices on U.S. Feedlots with a Capacity of Fewer than 1,000 Head.

Table 15. Percent of beef feedlot operations by nutrition management practice, by region, 2011

	Size of operation	
	Greater than 1,000 head	Less than 1,000 head
Percentage of feedlots		
Gave an ionophore, such as Rumesin© or Cattlyst©	90.5	28.7
Gave a coccidiostat other than an ionophore, such as Corid© or Deccox©	44.7	17.1
Percentage of cattle and calves		
Given an ionophore, such as Rumesin© or Cattlyst©	89.9	48.9
Given a coccidiostat other than an ionophore, such as Corid© or Deccox©	20.5	21.5

Source: USDA, Animal and Plant Health Inspection Service (APHIS), 2013a, pp. 51 and 52, Feedlot 2011 Part I: Management Practices on U.S. Feedlots with a Capacity of 1,000 or More Head. USDA, APHIS, 2013b, pp. 30 and 31, Feedlot 2011 Part II: Management Practices on U.S. Feedlots with a Capacity of Fewer than 1,000 Head.

In 2011, almost three-fourths of feedlots of 1,000 or more head administered antibiotics other than ionophores and coccidiostats in feed, accounting for 48 percent of cattle (Table 16; USDA, APHIS, 2013a). Only 26 percent of feedlots with less than 1,000 head did so, accounting for 38 percent of the head at these operations. Only 6 percent of large-scale feedlots that fed antibiotics (other than ionophores or coccidiostats) did so for more than 30 days (USDA, APHIS, 2013a).[13] Smaller scale feedlots that administered antibiotics were more likely to do so for longer than 30 days (20 percent of operations) (USDA, APHIS, 2013b). Note that with the statistics provided in the NAHMS publications, it is not possible to discern what percentages of these antibiotics were administered for growth promotion, disease prevention, or disease treatment. Statistics from an earlier 1994 NAHMS study of beef feedlots suggest that antibiotic use in feed and water has remained consistent since that year (USDA, APHIS, 2013c).

Table 16. Percentage of feedlots that gave an antibiotic in feed or water as a health- or production-management tool and percentage of cattle and calves receiving the antibiotics, 2011

	Size of operation	
	1,000 head or more	**Less than 1,000 head**
Percentage of feedlots giving antibiotics to at least some animals in…		
Feed	73.4	25.7
Water	4.7	1.5
Percentage of cattle and calves receiving antibiotics in…		
Feed	48.3	38.2
Water	0.3	7.6

Note: It is not possible from the statistics provided to discern the specific purpose of antibiotic administration (growth promotion or disease prevention).

Source: USDA, Animal and Plant Health Inspection Service (APHIS), 2013a, pp. 72 and 75, Feedlot 2011 Part I: Management Practices on U.S. Feedlots with a Capacity of 1,000 or More Head. USDA, APHIS, 2013b, pp. 36 and 37, Feedlot 2011 Part II: Management Practices on U.S. Feedlots with a Capacity of Fewer than 1,000 Head.

Dairy

How Is the U.S. Dairy Industry Structured?

Like other livestock industries, dairy production has shifted toward larger operations. Between 2000 and 2012, the share of production by farms with fewer than 100 head fell by half. A large number of small farms with dairy cows still exist, but these account for a small percentage of overall production. While over 70 percent of the 58,000 U.S. milk cow operations had fewer than 100 cows in 2012, these farms accounted for only 14 percent of milk production. Farms with milking herds of at least 1,000 head accounted for 51 percent of milk production but comprised only 3 percent of operations (USDA, NASS, 2013a).

In 2014, about 20 percent of dairy production occurred in California and another 20 percent in other Western States (Idaho, Washington, Oregon, Colorado, Arizona, and New Mexico). A further 20 percent took place in the upper-Midwestern States of Iowa, Minnesota, and Wisconsin. The Northeastern States New York, Pennsylvania, and Vermont were responsible for about 13 percent of milk production and the Eastern Corn Belt States Michigan, Indiana, and Ohio for about 10 percent (USDA, NASS, 2015).

Dairy farming differs from other livestock industries in important ways. First, most dairies do not operate under production contracts. Dairies usually market their milk through farmer-owned cooperatives to processors, but they may market to multiple firms or buyers. While compensation for their product varies with the attributes of the milk that they deliver to processors, dairy producers retain effective control over all major production decisions. There are a large number of dairy farms operating independently; hence, there are many decisionmakers for choices about antibiotic use.

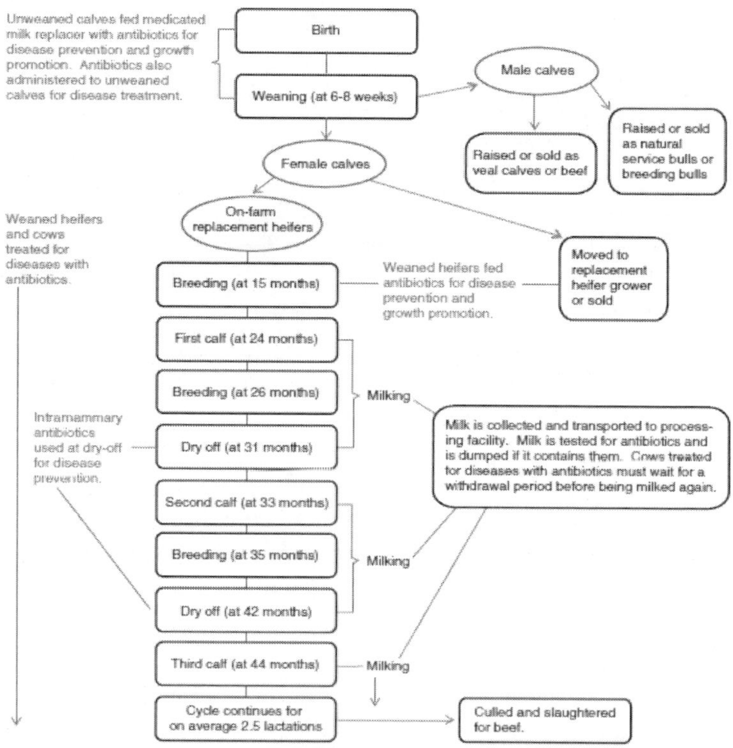

Source: USDA, Economic Research Service.

Figure 9. Dairy cow life cycle and use of antibiotics in stages of production.

Second, the nature of dairy production—in which birthing and milk production are intertwined— means that dairy farms combine lifecycle stages not usually combined in poultry, hog, and beef production (Figure 9). Farms rarely keep dairy bulls onsite, but instead rely largely on artificial insemination of cows with semen purchased from specialist providers. Milk cows typically give birth to calves on the dairy farm once a year and then provide milk for about 300 days before being "dried off" in preparation for the next calving. Male calves are usually sold immediately and raised for beef. Females are usually raised to be replacement heifers in the milking herd or sold to other dairy farms as replacement heifers. Heifers (milk cows that have not yet calved) are often raised onsite, but larger dairy farms may contract with specialist heifer-raising farms to take their calves and raise them until they are ready to enter the milking herd, at around 24 months of age. Heifers constitute approximately two-thirds of the milk cow herd (where the milk cow herd is inclusive of cows that have and have not calved).[14]

How Are Antibiotics Used in Dairy Production?

Antibiotics are used on dairy farms to treat and prevent disease, but they are also used in heifer rations for growth promotion. Diarrheal and respiratory problems are a large problem in preweaned dairy calves. Diarrhea and other digestive problems accounted for 56.5 percent of preweaned calf deaths at dairy farms in 2006, while respiratory problems accounted for 22.5 percent. In terms of morbidity, in 2006, 23.9 percent of unweaned dairy heifers on dairy operations were affected by a diarrheal or other digestive problem, while 12.4 percent were affected by a respiratory disease (Table 17).

To help prevent these illnesses and deaths, preweaned heifers are often fed medicated milk replacer that contains antibiotics. In 2006, 57.5 percent of dairy operations fed 49.9 percent of preweaned heifers medicated milk replacer. This practice was more common among small-and medium-sized dairy farms (fewer than 100 head and 100-499 head, respectively) than large dairy farms (500 or more head) (USDA, APHIS, 2007a). The most common medication in medicated milk replacer was oxytetracyline in combination with Neomycin (USDA, APHIS, 2007a). Dairy farms also use measures aside from antibiotics to reduce disease and disease transmission. Calves are often removed quickly from maternity pens in order to avoid nose-to-nose contact.

After a calf has been weaned at a dairy operation, respiratory problems account for a larger percentage of deaths (46.5 percent) than diarrheal deaths (12.6 percent). Weaned heifers may be fed coccidiostats and ionophores to prevent disease and promote growth. In 2006, 18.2 percent of dairy operators surveyed said that they included "antibiotics" in their heifer rations, while 32.7 percent stated they included ionophores (Table 18). Hence, at least half of dairies fed either antibiotics or ionophores to weaned heifers to prevent disease or promote growth. Cows at dairy operations may also be fed coccidiostats in

Table 17. Percentage of heifers and cows at dairy operations affected and treated with antibiotics for a disease or disorder during the previous 12 months, 2006

	Unweaned heifers			Weaned heifers			Cows		
	Percent of heifers		Percent of operations	Percent of heifers		Percent of operations	Percent of cows		Percent of operations
Disease or Disorder	Affected	Treated		Affected	Treated		Affected	Treated	
Respiratory	12.4	11.4	66.7	5.9	5.5	49.2	2.9	2.8	55.8
Diarrhea or other digestive problem	23.9	17.9	62.1	1.9	1.6	7.4	6.0	1.9	25.0
Navel infection	1.6	1.5	28.7						
Reproductive							10.0	7.4	52.9
Mastitis							18.2	16.4	85.4
Lameness							12.5	7.1	58.6
Other	0.6	0.6	4.5	1.7	1.4	6.2	0.7	0.5	6.9

Note: The percent of operations is the number of operations that used an antibiotic to treat the disease or disorder divided by all operations. It includes operations not reporting the occurrence of the disease or disorder. Shaded areas mean that the survey did not record the disease or disorder for the type of cow.

Source: USDA, Animal and Plant Health Inspection Service (APHIS) 2008, pp. 128, 129, 133, 134, 136, 137, Dairy 2007, Part III: Reference of Dairy Cattle Health and Management Practices in the United States, 2007.

Table 18. Percent of dairy operations by use of antibiotics in weaned-heifer rations to prevent disease or promote growth, 2006

	Percent operations
Antibiotics other than ionophores in heifer ration	18.2
Ionophores only in heifer rations	32.7
Did not know if antibiotics were in heifer ration	2.3
No antibiotics in heifer ration	44.2
No weaned heifers on operation	2.6

Source: USDA, Animal and Plant Health Inspection Service (APHIS), 2008, p. 131, Dairy 2007, Part III, Reference of Dairy Cattle Health and Management Practices in the United States, 2007.

feed to promote growth. In 2006, 26.8 percent of dairy operations fed 40 percent of dairy cows at these operations coccidiostats in feed (USDA, APHIS, 2007a).

After heifers are bred and give birth, they may contract diseases or disorders that are often treated with antibiotics. In 2006, 18.2 percent of cows were affected by mastitis, and 16.4 percent of cows were treated with antibiotics for mastitis (USDA, APHIS, 2008). Treated cows were located on 85.4 percent of operations (USDA, APHIS, 2008), suggesting that smaller operations were more likely to treat these diseases with antibiotics. Most dairy operations (90.1 percent) provide antibiotics for prevention of intramammary infections during the "dry" period (the time during which a cow is no longer milked in preparation for the next lactation) (USDA, APHIS, 2008).

Heifer-raising operations also include medications in feed to prevent disease and promote growth. In 2010, 77.3 percent of heifer operations (representing 87.3 percent of heifers at such operations) included ionophores in their weaned heifers' feed (Table 19). A full 87.1 percent of operations (92.4 percent of heifers) were fed some sort of medication to prevent disease or promote growth; among this group, the most often fed medications aside from ionophores were chlortetracycline compounds (27.8 percent of operations), coccidiostats (26.5 percent), and Aureomycin and sulfamethazine (25.6 percent).[15]

Table 19. Percentage of heifer-raising operations that used medicated feed in rations for weaned heifers to prevent disease or promote growth, 2010

Medication	Weaned heifers		Pregnant heifers	
	Percent operations	Percent heifers	Percent operations	Percent heifers
Ionophores	77.3	87.3	70.4	83.4
Coccidiostats	26.5	18.7	1.9	0.1
Chlortetracycline	27.8	23.8	7.9	5.6
Neomycin-oxytetracycline	1.4	10.9	0.0	0.0
Neomycin sulfate	1.4	8.8	0.0	0.0
Oxytetracycline compounds	9.0	1.0	3.7	1.8
Aureomycin and sulfamethazine	25.6	15.6	3.1	1.5
Tylosin sulfate	0.0	0.0	0.6	0.9
Other	2.4	1.8	1.2	2.0
Any medication	87.1	92.4	75.2	84.8
None	12.9	7.6	24.8	15.2

Source: USDA, Animal and Plant Health Inspection Service (APHIS), 2012, pp. 84, 85, 87, and 88, Dairy Heifer Raiser, 2011: An overview of operations that specialize in raising dairy heifers.

Research on the Economic Impacts of Use of Antibiotics for Production Purposes at the Animal and Farm Levels

This section focuses on the research methods used to estimate effects of antibiotics used for production purposes on animal and farm productivity, emphasizing how different methodologies may yield different results. The section then briefly discusses the varying sizes of effects in the broiler, hog, and cattle/dairy industries, given different research methods. More detailed discussion of individual research studies can be found in Appendix A.

Antibiotics are adopted because producers—whether farmer or integrator—think that they will reduce production costs per unit of meat. If widespread adoption lowers marketwide costs, producers will expand production, thereby lowering retail meat prices. In turn, lower prices will place pressure on producers who did not adopt antibiotics, while also inducing consumers to purchase more of the product. This set of economic impacts flows from the initial adoption decision, and, in turn, determines the likely economic impacts of antibiotic adoption or restriction. Understanding how use of production-purpose antibiotics affects animal and farm productivity is necessary for evaluating the potential market effects of restriction on use of antibiotics for such purposes. However, estimates of those effects vary widely, in large part because of differences in research methods and assumptions.

To understand how use of antibiotics for production purposes may affect livestock producer revenues, we first need to know how much their use affects animal productivity measures (production per animal) and how these productivity effects translate to changes at the farm level (costs per unit of output). As noted, animal-level productivity effects may have direct and indirect impacts at the level of the farm; costs of inputs (e.g., feed) may be directly affected by use of production-purpose antibiotics, but producers may adjust other inputs, as well as management practices, due to production-purpose antibiotic use or discontinuation, which may indirectly affect costs at the farm level.

Research Methods for Estimating Effects of Production-Purpose Antibiotic use on Productivity at the Animal and Farm Levels

Research on the animal- and farm-level productivity effects of production-purpose antibiotic use is based on *controlled experiments*, *observational studies* using cross-sectional comparisons of production, and examination of *outcomes after European bans on use of antibiotics for production purposes*. Other research uses the estimates of animal-level productivity effects from these three types of research to model farm-level outcomes. Table 20 provides basic descriptions of the research methods.

Controlled Experiments

In controlled experiments, researchers compare groups of identical animals, raised in identical environments except for the use of production-purpose antibiotics. One group receives the treatment (which could be either administration or discontinuation of production-purpose antibiotics, the 'treated' group), while the other does not (the 'control' group). Outcomes are compared for the treatment and control groups, and differences can be attributed to production-purpose antibiotics if the experimental design controls for all other factors affecting outcomes.

Observational Studies

Observational studies rely on survey data drawn from samples of operating farms. Some farms use production-purpose antibiotics while others do not, but in contrast to experimental studies, the two groups may also differ along other dimensions that affect outcomes (called confounding factors). Researchers can attempt to adjust for these differences via statistical methods. However, controlling for observable confounding factors does not always address selection bias—the fact that there are unobservable factors that cause especially productive or unproductive operations to use production- purpose antibiotics. For example, less efficient operations may choose to use production-purpose antibiotics in hope of improving outcomes, while more efficient operations may not. In that case, we may observe a negative relationship between production-purpose antibiotic use and outcomes, even if such use improves outcomes among those who adopt them, but this is not because production-purpose antibiotic use caused the negative outcome. Again, statistical methods can be used to at least partially correct for this selection issue. The ability to control for selection effects is limited by the fact that observational studies examining antibiotic outcomes use only one time period.

Research based on observational data may show smaller or larger effects of production-purpose antibiotic use than experimental studies. If production-purpose antibiotics are more effective in environments with poorer sanitation and worse management and are more likely to be adopted by producers with

Table 20. Types of studies used to estimate effects of use of antibiotics for production purposes

Type of study	Basic description	Possible limitations	Methods of overcoming these limitations to obtain effects of only production-purpose use of antibiotics
Experimental	Two groups are identical in every respect that can affect the outcome, except for the treatment (use of antibiotics for production purposes). One group receives antibiotics for production purposes while the other does not. Changes in the outcome can therefore be attributed to antibiotic use.	May not represent actual farm conditions. Does not represent how operations may alter practices in response to presence or absence of use of antibiotics for production purposes.	Examine actual farm conditions.
Observational, with survey data from one time period	Farm-level observations collected at one point in time. Farms using production-purpose antibiotics at that point compared to farms not using antibiotics for these purposes.	Correlations between production-purpose antibiotic use and outcomes may reflect other factors that are correlated with both outcomes and production- purpose antibiotic use. Outcomes may lead to changes in production-purpose antibiotic use, so correlations may reflect this direction of causality.	Control for factors correlated with both production-purpose antibiotic use and outcomes using statistical techniques. Statistical techniques can also be used to adjust for the effect of selection into production-purpose antibiotic use.
Observational, with survey data from before and after country-wide policy change in	Farm-level observations collected before and after country-wide changes in policy, usually a ban in production-purpose antibiotic	Operations may change other production practices when they can no longer use production-purpose antibiotics, so changes in outcomes may be attributable to both the change in production-	The goal of this research is to examine the effects of the bans, not necessarily the effects of just changes in production-purpose antibiotic use.

Type of study	Basic description	Possible limitations	Methods of overcoming these limitations to obtain effects of only production-purpose use of antibiotics
production-purpose antibiotic use ("ban research")	use. Outcomes compared before and after ban.	purpose antibiotic use and the other changes in production practices. Other factors affecting all farms that occur simultaneous to the ban may also impact outcomes.	
Modeled estimates of farm-level effects	Researcher generates a model of farm finances, using parameters from various sources. Effects of production-purpose antibiotics arise from other types of research.	Results dependent on the parameters chosen. If parameters for production-purpose antibiotic effects arise from experimental settings, results will not be inclusive of changes that producers may make in response to changing production-purpose antibiotic use. May assume that there are no other changes occurring in the market, which would not be the case in the event of industry-wide changes in production-purpose antibiotic use.	Depending on the scenario being modeled, researchers can include assumptions about changes at the market level. To model farm-level effects of production-purpose antibiotic use inclusive of alternative practices adopted in response to production-purpose antibiotic use changes, researchers can use parameter estimates of production-purpose antibiotic effects that include these other changes.

Source: USDA, Economic Research Service.

those environments, then their benefits and estimated effect sizes will be larger using observational data than effects found in experimental conditions. However, estimated effects may be smaller in actual production than in experimental studies because farm operators can adopt a number of methods to reduce the effect of not using antibiotics for production purposes.

Studies on Outcomes Following European Bans on use of Antibiotics for Production Purposes

A third line of research includes observational examinations of outcomes before and after a country-wide ban on use of antibiotics for production purposes, based on the series of bans introduced in European countries beginning in the 1980s. Because researchers do not control all variables influencing the outcomes, these studies are also considered observational. Note that when a country bans use of a drug for a specific purpose, there can be no comparisons of operations that still use the drug with similar operations (within the same country) that do not. Hence, if something else affects outcomes and happens at the same time as the ban, it is difficult for the researcher to separate the effect of the ban from that of the other occurrence. In these cases, researchers must carefully evaluate whether other factors that could be driving outcomes occurred simultaneously with the ban.

Research using bans to estimate effects may also show higher or lower effects of production-purpose antibiotics compared with controlled experiments for the same reasons described for comparing results from experimental research to those from survey data: effects in ban research may be higher because production units may be more poorly run than experimental farms. However, effect sizes may also be lower because other practices may be employed to reduce the effects of removing production-purpose antibiotic use. For example, if an operation must stop production-purpose antibiotic use and improves sanitation to help compensate, changes in outcomes may be the result of both actions. This also has a bearing on the profitability of producers: improving sanitation may lessen the effects that the ban has on animal growth rate but will likely add costs, which could reduce revenues if the ban is not accompanied by an increase in prices.

Studies Modeling Farm-Level Changes Based on Animal-Level Effects of Production- Purpose Antibiotics

Studies employing models of farm-level finances to estimate the impact of production-purpose antibiotic use or discontinuation generally use effects found in animal-level productivity research as parameters when estimating economic outcomes. For example, a finance study will take the effect of production-purpose antibiotic use on feed efficiency as reported in another study (say, a 2-percent increase) and multiply that by the price of feed to estimate the increased feed cost to a farmer if production-purpose antibiotic use is discontinued. This assumes that the farmer decided to produce the same amount of meat and did not alter other factors. Models that predict farm-level effects of production-purpose antibiotic use on profits or production often assume that the rest of the market remains static. For example, if stopping production-purpose antibiotic use increases production costs on individual farms and we assume nothing else changes, then revenue at individual farms will decline. However, if all farms stop using production-purpose antibiotics and supplies of meat decline as a result, this may increase meat prices for all farms. These higher prices may have a positive revenue effect. Consideration of just the farm-level effect in isolation from the market may provide estimates of short-term effects but not the entire story.

An important feature of all of these studies is the time period in which they were conducted. Management methods and industry structure have evolved in the livestock industry since the 1950s, with possible implications for the benefits of production-purpose antibiotics. For example, production-purpose antibiotics may produce larger outcomes in poultry houses with older management techniques or poor sanitation. As management methods have evolved over time, the effectiveness of production-purpose antibiotics may also have declined. The time period is also pertinent for farm-level models that use estimates of production-purpose antibiotic effects to predict changes in profits and productivity. Hence, it is useful to examine studies of production-purpose antibiotic productivity effects under current management regimes.

Animal- and Farm-Level Productivity Effects of Production-Purpose Antibiotics – Poultry

Although use of antibiotics for production purposes in broiler operations is common, research shows mixed effects on broiler productivity measures. Experimental research from the 1950s to the 1980s shows a wide range of effects, from negative to positive (see Appendix A). More recent experimental research reports small effects; researchers employed by Perdue Farms, Inc. (Engster, Marvil, and Stewart-Brown, 2002) found between a 0.14- and 0.2-percent reduction in mortality of chicks fed growth-promoting antibiotics and an average reduction of 0.016 pounds of feed per pound of live- weight gain (about 0.08 percent).

Observational research supports these findings of limited impacts of production-purpose antibiotic use on measures of broiler productivity. An observational study using nationally representative survey data compared broiler producers using antibiotics for purposes other than disease treatment with those using Hazard Analysis and Critical Control Points (HACCP) plans but not antibiotics for purposes other than disease treatment (MacDonald and Wang, 2011). Producers forgoing antibiotics except in the cases of disease treatment realized the same chick mortality, on average, as those feeding antibiotics for purposes other than disease treatment, while feed conversion was 2.5 percent higher (meaning more growth per unit of feed). The difference in feed conversion rose to 2.9 percent (in favor of antibiotics administered for purposes other than disease treatment) in a statistical model of production that controlled for other features of production. Estimated standard errors were large enough that a hypothesis of no-effect of antibiotics used for purposes other than disease treatment could not be rejected; the researchers note that producers forgoing antibiotics except in the case of disease treatment received higher contract fees, suggesting compensation for higher labor and capital costs associated with the higher sanitation methods of HACCP plans. Fees were approximately 2.1 percent higher for nonusers, suggesting a comparable increase in grower production costs, which in turn account for about 12.5 percent of producers' total costs, with integrators bearing the rest (MacDonald, 2014).

Research comparing outcomes before and after a country-wide ban on production-purpose antibiotics also found little change in productivity outcomes after removal of such antibiotic uses. Immediately after Denmark's 1998 ban on antimicrobial growth promoters, there was no significant change in mortality, but there was an increase of 0.016 pounds of feed per liveweight pounds produced (Emborg et al., 2001).

Animal- and Farm-Level Productivity Effects of Production-Purpose Antibiotics – Hogs

Like the findings for broilers, early experimental results for hogs show much larger effects than either later experimental studies or those employing survey data (see Appendix A). Experimental data before 1980 show large effects of production-purpose antibiotic use, including an increase in daily gain of 16.4 percent in young pigs and a 6.9 percent decline in the amount of feed required per unit of gain (Cromwell, 1991, citing research from 1950-1985). In finishing hogs, these effects were the same order of magnitude. Research from the 1980s and 1990s show smaller effects; a summary by Brorsen and coauthors (2002) finds a mean increase in feed efficiency of 2.74 percent in finishing hogs from production-purpose antibiotic use. A still later experimental study from 2002 finds that antimicrobials in feed have no effect on either growth promotion or feed efficiency of finishing hogs (Dritz et al., 2002). The authors do find a 5-percent increase in growth rate among nursery pigs associated with antimicrobials in feed, but no effect on feed efficiency. The lack of effects is attributed to greater sanitation in modern houses. Two recent studies on nursery pigs finds improved average daily growth and feed efficiency due to antibiotics: Oliver and Wells (2013) found a 5.4-percent increase, and Nemechek and coauthors (2014) found an approximately 9-percent increase, in average daily growth from feeding nursery pigs antibiotics.

Observational research that does not attempt to correct for selection biases (Miller et al., 2005; Liu, Miller, and McNamara, 2005) finds small, statistically significant effects of the use of antibiotics for growth promotion in finishing hogs. For a representative grower/finisher operation, growth-promoting antibiotics were predicted to improve average daily gain by 0.5 percent, while reducing feed conversion ratio by 1.1 percent and mortality by 0.22 percentage points.[16]

Observational studies that do account for selection bias find no statistically significant effects among finishing hogs in productivity, but some effects in nursery production (McBride, Key, and Mathews, 2008; Key and McBride, 2014). In a study that controls for the fact that producers make production decisions across many inputs, Key and McBride find a positive effect from growth-promoting antibiotics of 1 to 2 percent on the productivity at finishing hog facilities; however, this estimate is not statistically different from zero.

Research exploiting country-wide bans on antibiotics used for production purposes mainly shows small effects among nursery hogs (WHO, 2002). Effects are largest directly after the ban, but generally lessen over time. In Denmark's initial post-ban period, daily gain for weaner pigs declined by 5 percent and mortality increased by 0.7 percentage points (Kjeldsen, 2002). Reports on Sweden's ban suggest that effects on operations with good hygiene practices were minimal, and many producers converted to more modern production systems in response to the ban (Hayes et al., 1999).

Animal- and Farm-Level Productivity Effects of Production-Purpose Antibiotics – Beef and Dairy

Relative to broilers and hogs, there is little research examining the productivity effects of production-purpose antibiotics in beef and dairy cattle. Early experimental research on shows a wide range of effects, from positive to negative. Due to the range of outcomes, in the few instances where researchers attempt to estimate farm-level effects, they generally pick one experimental study's results and use this to predict changes at the farm level. Most research on effects of discontinuing use of production-purpose antibiotics in beef production examines market-level effects.

Summary of Animal- and Farm-Level Productivity Effects of Production- Purpose Antibiotics

Research on the effects of production-purpose antibiotics in animals and at the farm level shows a range of results. Older experimental research appears to show larger effects than newer research. More recent experimental research suggests that production-purpose antibiotics have small effects on broiler chick survival rates (less than 1 percent) and significant positive effects on the growth rate of nursery pigs (5 percent). Observational studies on hogs and broilers show small positive effects of production-purpose antibiotic use on mortality and feed efficiency, although the effects are often not statistically significant. In hogs, production-purpose antibiotics are associated with small increases (around 1 percent) in average daily gain and feed conversion rates for finishing hogs. Ban research suggests that production-purpose antibiotics increased the daily gain of young pigs by 5 percent.

Research suggests that farmers adopt alternative practices in order to increase productivity when they do not use production-purpose antibiotics. Observational research on broiler producers suggests that adopting a set of sanitation practices can mitigate any effects on feed efficiency of not using production-purpose antibiotics, but this is not without cost. The research also suggests that producers not using production-purpose antibiotics but using other practices have higher costs (by about 2 percent). Observational research on hog production shows the strongest effects of using production-purpose antibiotics among nursery hogs.

The small impacts found in the more recent literature suggest that policies to reduce production-purpose antibiotic use will not have large impacts on average farm-level productivity. The effects at the market level are also likely to be dampened because production-purpose antibiotic use is not universal. Despite the fact that these effects may not appear particularly large, production-purpose antibiotics are still widely administered in livestock production. Even with small effects, they may still be profitable choices. Estimated broiler feed costs came to 29 cents per liveweight pound produced in 2011 (MacDonald, 2014). With total liveweight production of 9.48 billion pounds, each 1-percent reduction in feed use would be worth $27.5 million to integrators, even if feed prices remained unchanged.

Effects at the farm level do not capture supply-chain adjustments resulting from production-purpose antibiotic restrictions. As described earlier, portions of the livestock lifecycle may occur in different settings. If production-purpose antibiotic restrictions disproportionately affect one portion, this may indirectly impact downstream portions. For example, if production-purpose antibiotic restrictions have a higher impact on nursery pigs than older hogs, this would affect the input supply to finishing operations. In another example, if production-purpose antibiotic restrictions increase the length of time to grow an animal to slaughter weight, processing facility timelines would be affected. Such effects will likely cause short-run adjustments, to be replaced with long-run modifications adapted to new production-purpose antibiotic restrictions.

EFFECTS OF PRODUCTION-PURPOSE ANTIBIOTIC USE AND DISCONTINUATION ON MARKET-LEVEL OUTCOMES

Restrictions on production-purpose antibiotic use will likely lead to small increases in production costs. Farmers and integrators will react to increased costs by changing production practices and by reducing production. In turn, reduced production will lead to price increases; consumers will react to increased prices by reducing consumption, and their response will affect the magnitude of the increase in prices, as well as lead to further changes to production, production costs, and seller profits. As a result of these market adjustments, the cost of restrictions will be borne in part by consumers through higher prices and in part by producers (integrators and farmers) through lower profits.

Market models help us understand how market prices and output are likely to change, as well as the impact of the policy change on different groups. While the prior sections have focused on the more detailed effects of restricting production-purpose antibiotic use in livestock production, this section examines effects on a broader, market-wide scale.

Supply and Demand in the Livestock Sector

To better understand the role of the market in determining price and output levels, we consider the supply and demand for meat (Figure 10). The supply curve shows the quantity that producers are willing and able to provide at each price, and the demand curve shows the quantity that consumers are willing and able to purchase at each price.

Research on the supply and demand for pork and chicken suggests these curves are inelastic, meaning that changes in price elicit less than proportionate changes in quantity demanded or supplied. An inelastic demand curve implies that if price rose by 1 percent, consumers would reduce purchases by less than 1 percent. An example of inelastic demand would be if the price of chicken breasts rose from $3 per pound to $3.03 per pound (a 1-percent increase) and consumers reduced purchases from 5 pounds to 4.98 pounds (a 0.04 percent decrease). Correspondingly, an inelastic supply means that if price rises by 1 percent, producers would be willing to supply less than 1 percent more of the good.

If production-purpose antibiotic use were limited, then it would be more expensive to produce each unit of the good, and suppliers would require a higher price for each unit provided. The supply curve would shift to the left (from Supply to Supply' in Figure 10), and suppliers would produce less at the original price P_0. A smaller supply would drive prices upward, and higher prices would cause consumers to move along the demand curve and purchase less meat. Market prices would then be driven to a price (P_2) that again equates demand and supply in the market, now at a quantity Q_2. Consumers would be consuming less and paying more, and producers would be receiving higher prices but producing less. Producers' total revenue (P multiplied by Q) may increase if the decline in production is outweighed by the increase in price.

Given how suppliers behave (as represented by Supply and Supply'), the size of the price increase and quantity decline will depend on the price elasticity of demand. If the demand curve were much steeper (more inelastic), so that consumers were less responsive to price changes, price would rise by more, and quantity would fall by less, than is depicted in Figure 10. Alternatively, if consumers were quite responsive to price changes, so that the

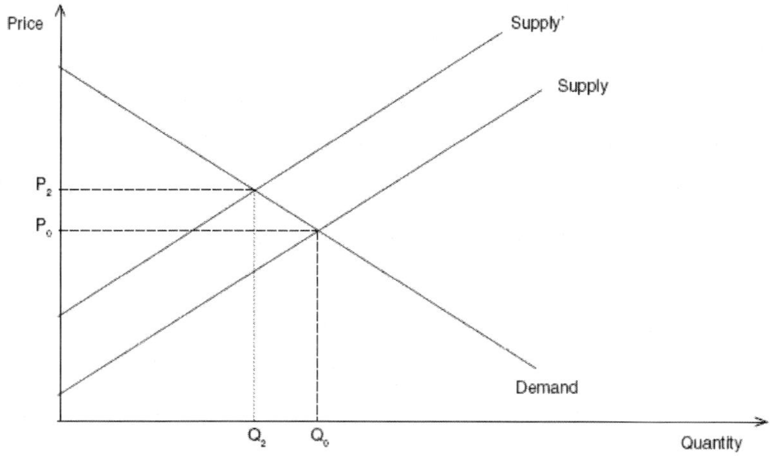

Source: USDA, Economic Research Service.

Figure 10. Supply and demand for meat.

demand curve was much flatter, then price would rise by less but quantity would fall considerably.

The effects of a ban will be felt differently by producers more reliant on production-purpose antibiotics and those who are less so. In the beginning of a ban, producers less reliant on production-purpose antibiotics would experience less of an increase in their costs of production and would gain profits. Those who did not use production-purpose antibiotics before the ban may even increase production in response to higher prices. Producers more reliant on production-purpose antibiotics would experience a greater increase in their costs of production and would lower quantity produced. Some may even exit the industry.

Research on Market-Level Effects of Reductions in Production-Purpose Antibiotic Use

To examine the likely market-level effects of restrictions on production-purpose antibiotic use, a researcher must develop a model of the livestock industry, with components representing the effect of restrictions on production costs and the share of production that is affected by the restrictions (the supply shift), how the total supply of meat relates to price (including the price elasticity of supply), and how much demand for meat there is at each price (including the price elasticity of demand). This type of research must, by necessity, make many assumptions on how an entire market would function. Different models will incorporate different assumptions and may or may not allow other features to change in response to a production-purpose antibiotic reduction.

Prior research performing this type of analysis universally assumes that production costs increase due to production-purpose antibiotic restrictions, yielding a reduction in supply. Short descriptions of these studies are provided in Appendix A; all are long studies that analyze several scenarios and make different assumptions, so it is difficult to succinctly compare them. Notably, the largest estimated losses occur in research published before 1980 that rely on production-purpose antibiotic effect sizes at the animal level from earlier experimental research.

These studies all rely on estimated effects at the animal level of reducing production-purpose antibiotic use, as discussed above. In all research except for Hayes and coauthors (1999), the authors use effect sizes from early experimental research conducted before 1980. As noted, the effect sizes found in experimental research can overestimate what happens in actual farm conditions when production-purpose antibiotic use is restricted. Hence, the effects of production-purpose antibiotic restrictions may be much more limited than the early experimental literature would suggest, although not without some costs.

Hayes and coauthors (1999 and 2001) are the only researchers to generate estimates of the effects of production-purpose antibiotic restrictions on producer and consumer surplus using effect sizes from the ban research. The ban research examines what actually happened when countries banned or limited production-purpose antibiotic use in livestock production; the effect sizes thus include farmers' adaptations to production-purpose antibiotic restrictions.

Estimating Changes in Market-Level Outcomes from Production-Purpose Uses of Antibiotics

None of the prior studies employ effect sizes of production-purpose antibiotic use that arise from observational data from the United States. To estimate market-wide effects of reducing production- purpose antibiotic use, we use the effect sizes from observational studies by Key and McBride (2014) and MacDonald and Wang (2011) in a basic model of the U.S. markets for pork and broilers. Because these studies use production function methods, how the results factor into a model will differ somewhat from prior studies. As a starting point, prior studies use effects on one or two particular inputs. For example, a study might use the effect of production-purpose antibiotics on feed efficiency to estimate how much more feed would be needed to produce the same amount of meat, but it would not account for how other facets of production might change in response to production-purpose antibiotic restrictions.

Unlike these prior studies, Key and McBride (2014) and MacDonald and Wang (2011) account for many inputs, reflecting the fact that producers make a number of production decisions about input levels, as well as about management techniques. The results can therefore be interpreted as percent changes in production, holding prices constant, from adjusting other inputs while forgoing production-purpose antibiotics.

As described above, at the market level, if production were to become more costly at each price, the supply would decrease, leading to a lower level of overall production as well as higher prices. To estimate various effects at the market level, we make assumptions about several market parameters and then estimate effects under different scenarios, using Monte Carlo simulation.[17] This type of analysis enables the researchers to assess the range of possible outcomes, given multiple uncertain parameters, including the supply-change effect of a ban, the percentage of producers using production-purpose antibiotics before the ban, and the elasticities of the supply and demand curves.

Our supply-change ranges are based on Key and McBride and MacDonald and Wang. Key and McBride find a 1- to 1.3-percent increase in productivity if antibiotics for growth promotion are used in feeder-to-finish hog operations, but note that this result is not statistically significant. They also show that antibiotics used for growth promotion reduced deviations in unexplained output by 1.4 percent. MacDonald and Wang found that users of antibiotics for purposes other than disease treatment (inclusive of antibiotics for both growth promotion and disease prevention) consumed 2.5 percent less feed per pound of liveweight production than nonusers with HACCP plans and 4 percent less than other nonusers. More complete models of production placed the effects at 3 percent greater output, given all inputs, although the estimates were not statistically different from zero (the researchers could not reject the hypothesis that there was no effect). Hence, as lower and upper bounds, we use effect sizes of 1 and 3 percent. Because the results are from Key and McBride and

MacDonald and Wang are not statistically discernible from no effect, however, it is possible that production-purpose antibiotic restrictions will have no effect on market prices or volumes.

Experimental results from Dritz and coauthors (2002) and Nemechek and coauthors (2013) suggest that production-purpose antibiotics only affect young hogs, with an approximate 5-percent effect size. We examine a different scenario in which a production-purpose antibiotic ban would only affect nursery hogs, with supply changes ranging from 4 to 6 percent. Since nursery hogs constitute only 22 percent of production, the effects on the entire hog sector are limited.

As noted, not all livestock are administered production-purpose antibiotics. Hence, restrictions on production-purpose antibiotic use would only impact a portion of producers, and the overall impact on the market of restrictions would be lessened. Using ARMS data, we estimate that between 36 and 59 percent of hog production involves antibiotics for growth promotion and that antibiotics are used in 20 to 52 percent of broiler production. For a third scenario, in which production-purpose antibiotic restrictions only impact nursery pigs, we calculate that only 22 percent of hog production occurs in the nursery stage and that only 23 to 49 percent of nursery hogs receive growth-promoting antibiotics. In this scenario, therefore, only 23 to 49 percent of 22 percent of production is affected. Further parameters used in the model, along with their sources, are shown in Table 21. See Appendix B for further description of the model.

The results of the simulation assuming a 1- to 3-percent change in supply show reductions in output of less than 0.5 percent for pork and chicken (Table 22). Wholesale prices increase by 0.77 percent for pork and 0.73 percent for chicken. Prices rise more than output declines, yielding greater total revenue for pork and broiler producers (0.29 percent for pork and 0.42 percent for chicken).

As described above, we perform many simulations to generate the range in possible outcomes at the market level. Figures 11 and 12 show the distribution of simulation outcomes for the pork and broiler markets, assuming a 1- to 3-percent supply change. Ninety-five percent of simulations yield a pork wholesale price change of between 0.20 and 1.2 percent. For changes in pork production, 95 percent of simulations show declines between 0.85 and 0.10 percent. Only 5 percent of simulations suggest declines in total revenue, while 90 percent yield increases in total revenue between zero and about 0.6 percent.

Table 21. Model assumptions

Parameter	Value(s)	Source(s)	Notes
Hogs			
Elasticity of supply	Mean: .65 Standard deviation: 0.163	Muth et al., 2007	Standard deviation set at 25% of mean; assumed normally distributed
Elasticity of demand	Mean: -0.635 Standard deviation: 0.159	Muth et al., 2007	Standard deviation set at 25% of mean; assumed normally distributed.
Baseline production (million lb) (2012)	23,270	USDA, 2014a	
Baseline wholesale price ($/lb) (2012)	1.47	USDA, 2014b	
Percentage of production value in nursery hogs	0.22	Calculations from ARMS 2009 data	
Percentage of all production receiving antibiotics	Minimum: 0.36 Maximum: 0.59	Calculations from ARMS 2009 data	Percentage of hogs sold or removed receiving antibiotics via feed or water for growth promotion. Values for nursery and finish hogs were combined according to the percentage of production value in nursery hogs. Assumed uniformly distributed between minimum and maximum.
Percentage of young hogs receiving antibiotics	Minimum: 0.23 Maximum: 0.49	Calculations from Agricultural Resource Management Survey 2009 data	Percentage of hogs sold or removed receiving antibiotics via feed or water for growth promotion. Assumed uniformly distributed between minimum and maximum.
Percentage change in supply from production-purpose antibiotic restrictions - - all hogs	Minimum: 0.01 Maximum: 0.03	See summaries of past research.	Assumed uniformly distributed between minimum and maximum.
Percentage change in supply from production-purpose antibiotic restrictions - - just nursery hogs	Minimum: 0.04 Maximum: 0.06		
Broilers			
Elasticity of supply	Mean: 0.59 Standard deviation: 0.148	Holt and Aradhyula, 1990	Standard deviation set at 25% of mean; assumed normally distributed.

Table 21. Model assumptions (Continued)

Parameter	Value(s)	Source(s)	Notes
Elasticity of demand	Mean: -0.43 Standard deviation: 0.108	Muth et al., 2006	Standard deviation set at 25% of mean; assumed normally distributed.
Baseline production (million lb) (2012)	36,643	USDA, 2014c	
Baseline wholesale price ($/lb) (2012)	0.85	USDA, 2014d	
Percentage of production receiving antibiotics	Minimum: 0.20 Maximum: 0.52	Calculations from ARMS 2011	Percentage of production receiving antibiotics for purposes other than illness. Assumed uniformly distributed between minimum and maximum.
Percentage change in supply from restrictions in use of production-purpose antibiotics	Minimum: 0.01 Maximum: 0.03	See summaries of past research.	Assumed uniformly distributed between minimum and maximum.

Source: USDA, Economic Research Service. ARMS = Agricultural Resource Management Survey.

Table 22. Market-level effects of full ban on antibiotic use for production purposes in hogs and broilers, Monte Carlo estimation results

	Scenario		
	-3% reduction in supply from limiting production uses of antibiotics		**4-6% effect on young pig productivity from limiting production uses of antibiotics**
	Hogs	**Broilers**	**Hogs**
% Change in output	-0.47	-0.31	-0.20
	(0.18)	(0.14)	(0.06)
% Change in wholesale price	0.77	0.73	0.32
	(0.30)	(0.33)	(0.10)
% Change in value of production	0.29	0.42	0.12
	(0.20)	(0.23)	(0.08)
% Change in output, producers not using antibiotics for production purposes	0.48	0.42	0.20
	(0.18)	(0.18)	(0.06)
% Change in output, producers using antibiotics for production purposes	-1.53	-1.59	-4.81
	(0.46)	(0.48)	(0.55)

% Change in value of production, producers not using antibiotics for production purposes	0.28 (0.21)	0.31 (0.22)	0.12 (0.08)
% Change in value of production, producers using antibiotics for production purposes	-0.77 (0.35)	-0.87 (0.43)	-4.50 (0.54)

Note: Standard deviations shown in parentheses.
Source: USDA, Economic Research Service, authors' estimates.

The distributions of simulation outcomes in the chicken market are similarly narrow. In 95 percent of simulations, the increase in price is between 0.1 and 1.3 percent. Ninety-five percent of simulations yield declines in quantity produced between 0.6 and 0.05 percent. No simulations suggest declines in broiler total revenues; 95 percent of simulations suggest increases between 0.05 and 0.75 percent.

While the change in total industry revenue is positive, the effect on producers depends on whether they used production-purpose antibiotics before the ban. With lower farm productivity, production- purpose antibiotic users would reduce output by about 1.53 percent in pork and 1.59 percent in broilers, while higher prices would induce nonusers to increase output by 0.48 percent for pork and 0.42 percent for chicken. While production declines for users, the accompanying price increase mitigates the effect to an extent such that users see a decreased value of revenue of less than 1 percent (0.77 percent for pork and 0.87 percent for chicken). Nonusers see small increases in revenue (0.28 percent for pork and 0.31 percent for chicken).

When restrictions on production-purpose antibiotic use affect only nursery hogs, we generally see smaller impacts at the market level because only a small share of the market is being affected. The only outcome for which there is a larger effect is in the change of output of producers using production-purpose antibiotics. Because only a small share of the market both raises nursery hogs and uses production-purpose antibiotics, the effect of the supply decrease is concentrated among these users; they see a 4.81-percent reduction in output and a decrease in total value of production of 4.5 percent.

Note that the simulation estimates average effects at the level of the market, not effects for individual producers. Individual producers may see effects of production-purpose antibiotic restrictions that are smaller or larger than the predicted market changes.

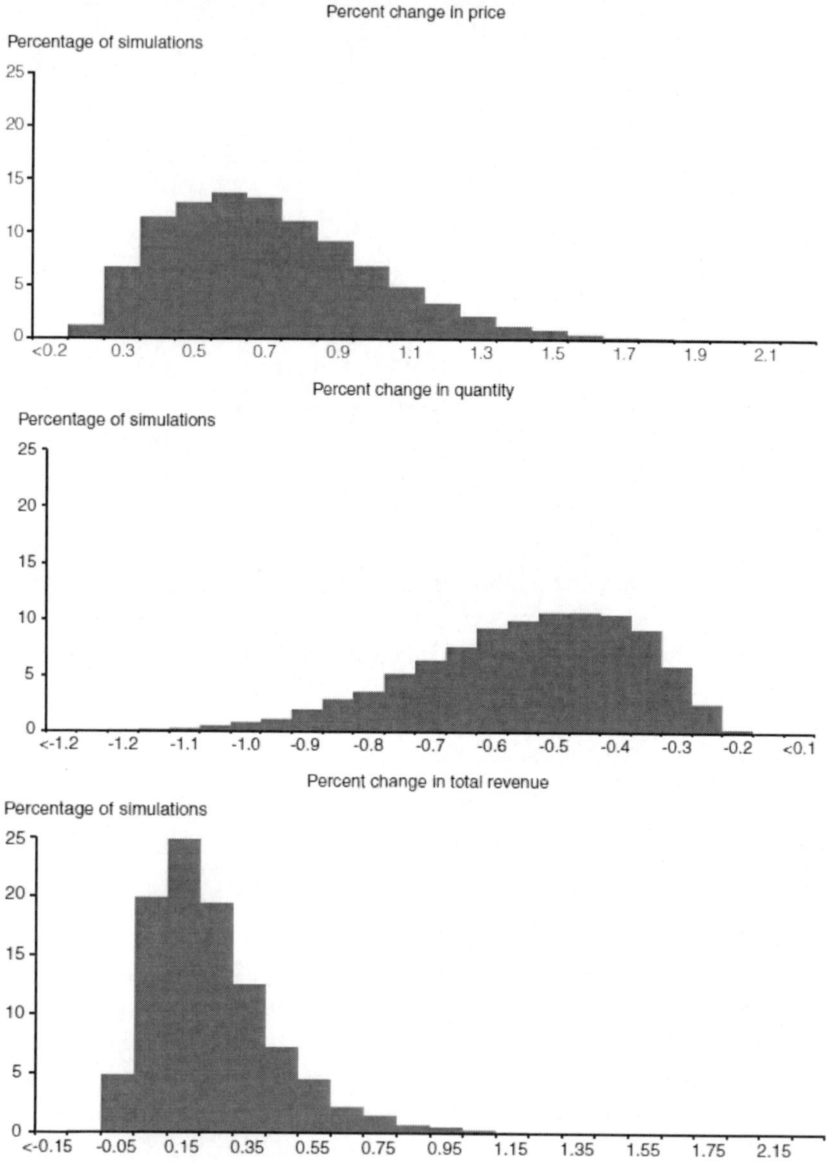

Source: USDA, Economic Research Service.

Figure 11. Distribution of simulation outcomes for the pork market.

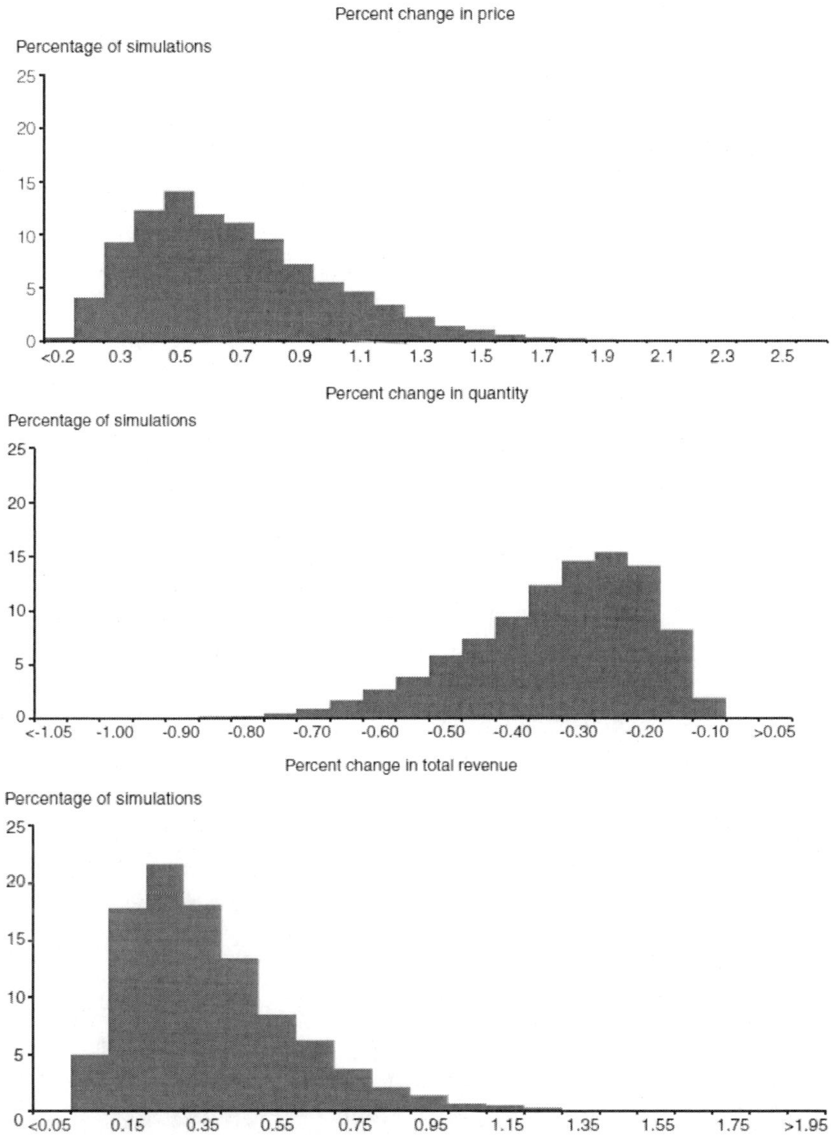

Source: USDA, Economic Research Service.

Figure 12. Distribution of simulation outcomes for the chicken market.

Limitations to the Market Model

While this simple model provides useful information about the order of magnitude of effects of restrictions on production-purpose antibiotic use, it relies on a number of simplifying assumptions and overlooks several features of the market, as well as some effects of the ban.

Recent FDA actions to reduce production uses of antimicrobials in livestock agriculture only target drugs that are important to human medicine. However, the estimated effect sizes from MacDonald and Wang and Key and McBride examine use of *any* antibiotics for production purposes. Thus if only some antibiotics were restricted for use in livestock production, the impact would be smaller than the 1- to 3-percent those authors found. Additionally, MacDonald and Wang estimate productivity effects for both disease prevention and production purposes. Because the FDA actions only restrict production purposes, the impacts estimated in the market model for the broiler sector are likely larger than those from restrictions mirroring current FDA ones.

The model does not examine changes in associated industries. For example, the restrictions are likely to affect feed use in the broiler and hog industries, as the loss of growth-promoting antibiotics leads to increased feed consumption per animal, offset to some extent by a decline in total production. This may have repercussions in the grain sector, which is not analyzed. Additional sectors that are not examined but that might experience repercussions from a ban are the pharmaceutical and veterinary industries.

In this simulation, the only policy examined is a ban on use of antibiotics used for production purposes. It does not examine effects of requiring veterinary prescriptions for drugs previously available over the counter; the FDA is currently taking such an action with Guidance 213 (U.S. FDA, 2013). As noted in the discussion on industry structure, the geographic concentration and level of vertical integration will likely impact the implementation and costs of meeting this new requirement. The model uses estimates of supply elasticities based on short- and intermediate-term responses to price changes over 1 to 12 quarters. This time horizon coincides with the FDA's proposed approach of having drug sponsors voluntarily remove production purposes as labeled uses for medically important antimicrobials within a 3-year period. Over longer periods, producers have more margins for adjustments—for instance, by altering the size of breeding populations and constructing new facilities or closing existing ones—and long-run supply elasticities may therefore be considerably larger. The model is also not directly comparable to the studies that examine what would happen in a single quarter after a ban.

While production-purpose antibiotics can increase productivity and lower prices of meat production, another economic aspect of their use includes potential shifts in the demand curve (rather than movements along it). Consumers may demand products raised without antibiotics, and individual consumer demand may also be represented by large-scale retailers. In the event that consumers have a wide-scale preference for meat raised without production-purpose antibiotics and policy changes mean that meat is raised with fewer production-purpose antibiotics, consumers may demand more meat, potentially by substituting out of other foods. This would lead to a rightward shift in the demand curve (not shown in Figure 10). The model also does not account for substitution between types of meat. If production-purpose antibiotic restrictions were to impact one type of livestock production more than another, then prices could increase unevenly, leading consumers to substitute between meat types.

Finally, these analyses focus entirely on the costs of restrictions and how they fall on groups of producers and consumers. They do not focus on any human or animal health benefits derived from reduced use of antibiotics.

CONCLUSION

The use of antibiotics in livestock agriculture is a contested topic, and recent Federal guidelines have been adopted to reduce the practice. However, recent statistics from multiple, nationally representative surveys suggest that antibiotic use for growth promotion is not universal and in some industries is declining. This may be because the efficacy of antibiotics in increasing farm-level productivity has decreased, as suggested by both experimental and observational research published since 2000. This research shows that antibiotics used for production purposes generally have limited effects on the productivity of raising livestock at the farm level (at most, on the order of 1 to 3 percent). Given that only a portion of producers use antibiotics for production purposes and that on average their use appears to have little impact, restrictions are predicted to change prices and quantities by less than 1 percent over time. Like European countries that have stopped using growth-promoting antimicrobials, U.S. producers are likely to adopt alternative practices in place of antibiotics for production purposes.

Appendix A: Prior Research on the Effects of Using Antibiotics for Production Purposes at the Animal, Farm, and Market Levels

Animal-Level Productivity Effects of the Use of Antibiotics for Production Purposes in Broilers

Experimental research on the animal-level effects of use of antibiotics for production purposes in broiler outcomes shows widely varying effects (Table A1). Research from the 1950s through the 1980s shows mixed results of the effect of production-purpose antibiotics in poultry growth (see Emborg et al., 2001, for an overview). Results vary according to the type of antibiotic or combination of antibiotics fed. Effects range from none at all to a 19-percent increase in average body weight and an 8-percent increase in feed conversion. A 1981 report summarizing research that is largely from the 1950s through 1970s suggests growth effects of different antibiotics between negative 3.3 percent to positive 16 percent, with most antibiotics showing positive effects (CAST, 1981).

More recent experimental research shows very small effects of use of antibiotics for production purposes. Engster, Marvil, and Stewart-Brown (2002) compared production outcomes in 158 paired poultry production houses in North Carolina and the Delmarva Peninsula. The authors were researchers employed by Perdue Farms, Inc., one of the leading poultry producers in the United States. Trial and control houses were paired on the same farm. Trial houses used no growth- promoting antibiotics, while control houses continued to use them; otherwise, each paired house was the same size, with identical technologies, production practices, chick placements, and cycle lengths. Feed conversion rates for birds fed growth-promoting antibiotics were higher in trial houses in each trial period and location, but the average difference was less than a 1-percent increase. Flocks receiving growth-promoting antibiotics had a lower percentage of chicks surviving, by 0.2 percent in the Delmarva Peninsula and 0.14 percent in North Carolina. Another finding of this analysis suggests that the effectiveness of growth-promoting antibiotics may be conditional on sanitary practices; after a full house clean-out, houses *not* receiving growth-promoting antibiotics had *higher* livability and *higher* weight gain per unit feed than control houses. These effects deteriorated in subsequent flocks placed in the same houses without litter removal. Unfortunately, the authors report only differences in means in the outcomes, not whether they were statistically significantly different. Hence, it isn't possible to know whether growth-promoting antibiotics led to any difference in outcomes in this study.

A second type of research examining the effects of use of production-purpose antibiotics on animal outcomes uses observational data from large surveys. For poultry, the most recent research on effectiveness of antibiotics used for purposes other than disease treatment in broiler operations examines Agricultural and Resource Management Survey (ARMS) data. MacDonald and Wang (2011) use nationally representative 2006 ARMS data on broiler producers that use antibiotics for disease prevention and/or growth promotion and those that do not. They find that producers using antibiotics only for disease treatment employ a distinctly different set of production practices from those that do. One such difference is the use of a Hazard Analysis and Critical Control Points (HACCP) plan; compared to producers using antibiotics for non-disease-treatment reasons, producers using HACCP plans but not non-disease-treatment antibiotics were more likely to test flocks for pathogens, use all-in all-out production, have new buildings, and institute a number of other sanitation methods. Comparing producers stating that they use antibiotics for purposes other than disease treatment with those that do not but do use a HACCP plan, MacDonald and Wang found no statistically significant difference in the feed conversion rate. The research indicates that if use of antibiotics for purposes other than disease treatment was banned, growers could adapt without declines in production. However, the researchers note that producers using antibiotics only for disease treatment purposes received higher contract fees, suggesting compensation for the higher labor and capital costs associated with the more thorough sanitation methods of HACCP plans. Fees were approximately 2.1 percent higher for producers only using antibiotics for disease treatment (not growth promotion or disease prevention), suggesting a comparable increase in production costs.

Turning to studies using country-wide bans, Emborg and coauthors (2001) examined the effects on poultry outcomes of Denmark's ban on antimicrobial growth promoters by comparing flocks slaughtered before and after the 1998 ban. They found no significant change in mortality rates after the ban, nor did they find a significant change in capacity utilization (broiler production per square meter). However, directly after the ban, they did find a statistically significant increase of 0.016 pounds of feed per liveweight pounds produced (a reduction in feed efficiency). This effect remained until the end of the study period 16 months after the ban.

Examination of Sweden's 1986 ban on antimicrobial growth promoters by Wierup (2001) focuses specifically on changing production practices due to the ban. He notes that producers altered feed rations as well as improving sanitation and ventilation in houses. Based on these changes, along with an initial increase in antibiotics administered at doses for disease treatment, Weirup suggests that any problems associated with the ban were prevented.

Farm-Level Productivity Effects of Production-Purpose Antibiotics – Poultry

Even if production-purpose antibiotics have beneficial effects on feed efficiency, growth, and other animal health markers, they may not be economically efficient if the costs of production-purpose antibiotics outweigh the benefits. Graham, Boland, and Silbergeld (2007) examine this question. They first note the results from Engster, Marvil, and Stewart-Brown (2002, described above) on the effects of using growth-promoting antibiotics on mortality, average weight, condemnations (rejected for human consumption), and feed-conversion ratios. They then estimate the change in payment to the grower and the cost to produce broilers, assuming specific parameters for the cost of feed, the cost of antibiotics, and payment rates to growers per pound of chicken, as well as starting values for mortality rate, condemnation rate, feed conversion ratio, and average weight. The researchers find a net effect of growth-promoting antibiotic use to producers of *negative* \$0.0093 per chick (or 0.45 percent of total cost), suggesting that the costs of production-purpose antibiotics were greater than the benefits in terms of lower mortality rates and greater feed efficiency. However, Graham, Boland, and Silbergeld apparently value broilers at the fee paid to the grower (about 5 cents per pound) rather than at the value of the bird to the integrator (40 or 50 cents per pound). Also note that these estimates do not take account of a variety of factors about market-level effects, as well as effects in other portions of the industry.

Lawson, Jensen, and Otto (2008) construct production functions for poultry production facilities and compare how inputs were used differently before and after Denmark's 1999 ban on antimicrobial growth promoters. They find that by substituting between inputs, poultry producers can maintain their production amounts in the absence of antibiotics for growth promotion.

Animal-Level Productivity Effects of Production-Purpose Antibiotics – Hogs

Research on production-purpose antibiotic effects on hog productivity differentiates by phase of production. Table A2 summarizes research of production-purpose antibiotic effects on animal- and farm-level outcomes. Earlier experimental results show much larger effects than either later experimental studies or those employing survey data. Cromwell (1991) summarizes experimental research performed between 1950 and 1985. He notes that for that period, the use of production- purpose antibiotics in young pigs improved growth rate by an average of 16.4 percent and reduced the amount of food required by pound of gain (feed efficiency) by 6.9 percent. The effect of production-purpose antibiotics in the grower/finisher phase was lower than in young pigs: a gain of 4.2 percent in growth rate and 2.2 percent in feed efficiency. Cromwell also compares studies from 1950 to 1977 to those for 1978 to 1985 to suggest that effect sizes declined minimally, if at all, from the first period to the second.

Appendix Table A1. Summary of literature on effects of production-purpose antibiotic use and discontinuation on animal- and farm-level outcomes in poultry

Source	Time of study	Type of study	Outcome	Effect size of production-purpose antibiotic use
CAST, 1981	1950s	Review of experimental studies	Feed conversion	Production-purpose antibiotics increase feed conversion by 8%
			Growth	Production-purpose antibiotics decrease growth by as much as 3.3% or increase it by as much as 16%
Engster, Marvil, and Stewart-Brown, 2002	2002	Experimental study of removing growth-promoting antibiotics	Feed conversion	0.012 lb feed/lb body weight gain increase (0.8% increase)[b]
			Percentage of chicks surviving	0.2% decline
			Bodyweight	Decline of 0.041[b] (0.8%

				decline)[c]
Graham, Boland, and Silbergeld, 2007	2002	Farm-level model of value from using growth-promoting antibiotics	Value per chicken	Decrease from using production purpose antibiotics of \$0.012/chicken (2013\$)[a]
MacDonald and Wang, 2011	2006	Observational using one period of survey data, comparing producers using antibiotics for purposes other than disease treatment and those not using antibiotics for purposes other than disease treatment but using a HACCP plan	Feed conversion	No statistically significant difference
			Contract fees	2.1% higher in producers foregoing use of antibiotics for growth promotion or disease prevention
Emborg et al., 2001	Before and after 1998	Observational, using survey data collected before and after Denmark's ban on antimicrobial growth-promoters	Mortality rate	No statistically significant change after ban
			Capacity utilization	No statistically significant change after ban
			Pounds of feed per live-weight produced	0.016 pound increase after ban

[a] Graham, Boland, and Silbergeld (2002) report a value of \$0.0093. This was updated to 2013 dollars using the Consumer Price Index.

[b] Assuming a feed conversion rate of 1.96 to estimate percentage difference.

[c] Assuming a final bodyweight of 5 lb to estimate percentage difference.

Source: Compiled by USDA, Economic Research Service from literature survey.

Appendix Table A2. Summary of literature on effects of production-purpose antibiotic use and discontinuation on animal- and farm-level outcomes in hogs

Source	Time of study	Type of study	Outcome	Effect size of production-purpose antibiotic use or discontinuation
Cromwell, 1991	1950-1985	Summary of experimental studies	Daily gain, young pigs	16.4% (effect of use)
			Feed/gain, young pigs	-6.9% (effect of use)
			Daily gain, growing phase	10.6% (effect of use)
			Feed/gain, growing phase	-4.5% (effect of use)
			Daily gain, grower/finisher pigs	4.2% (effect of use)
			Feed/gain, young pigs	-2.2% (effect of use)
Robertsson and Lend-eheim, 1994	Before and after 1986	Observational study surveying a set of farms before and after Sweden's 1986 ban	Post-weaning piglet mortality	0.4-0.5 percentage point increase (effect of discontinuing use)
			Number of pigs weaned/litter	4.9% (effect of use)[a]
			Percentage piglets surviving until weaning	1.7 percentage points (effect of use)[a]
			Percentage of breeding pigs that farrowed	7 percentage points (effect of use)
Cromwell, 2002	Studies largely from the 1960s	Summary of experimental studies	Live pigs born per litter	3.0% (effect of use)[a]
			Number of pigs weaned/litter	4.9% (effect of use)[a]
			Percentage piglets surviving until weaning	1.7 percentage points (effect of use)[a]
			Percentage of breeding pigs that farrowed	7 percentage points (effect of use)

Source	Time of study	Type of study	Outcome	Effect size of production-purpose antibiotic use or discontinuation
Dritz, Tokach, Goodband, and Nelssen, 2002	Before 2002	Experimental study	Growth rate, nursery pigs	5% (effect of use)
			Growth rate, finishing pigs	No statistically significant effect (effect of use)
			Feed efficiency, nursery pigs and finishing pigs	No statistically significant effect (effect of use)
Brorsen et al., 2002	Studies from 1980s and 1990s	Summaries of scientific studies	Feed efficiency, finishing pigs	-1% to 5% (effect of use), average of 2.74%
			Mortality reduction, finishing pigs	0.75 percentage points
			Sort loss reduction	\$0.60/hog (effect of use)[b]
	Simulation	Benefit per hog	\$3.59/hog (effect of use)[b]	
World Health Organization (WHO), 2002 citing Larsen, 2002	Before and after 1998	Observational study using data from before and after	Number of antibiotic treatments	Increased from 0.4 per pig-month to 1.0 per pig-month (effect of discontinuing use)
			Incidence of diarrhea treatment in finisher hogs	Initial increase but return to pre-ban levels within 1 year (effect of discontinuing use)
Kjeldsen, 2002	Before and after 1998	Observational study using survey data from before and after Sweden's national ban	'Permanent' problems like reduced daily gain or increased diarrhea treatments	11% of herds showed problems (effect of discontinuing use)
			Mortality rate of finisher hogs	0.2 percentage point increase (effect of discontinuing use)
			Daily gain of weaner pigs	5% decline (effect of discontinuing use)
			Mortality of weaner pigs	0.7 percentage point increase (effect of discontinuing use)
			Length of time for weaner pigs to reach 30kg	3% increase (effect of discontinuing use)

Appendix Table A2. (Continued)

Source	Time of study	Type of study	Outcome	Effect size of production-purpose antibiotic use or discontinuation
Miller et al., 2003	1990 and 1995	Observational study using survey data	Average daily gain	0.5% (effect of use)
			Feed conversion ratio	1.1% (effect of use)
			Profits	$0.75 per pig marketed (effect of use)[c]
			Mortality rate	-0.22 percentage points (effect of use)
Dibner and Richards, 2005, citing Callesen, 2003	1995-1998 and 1999-2001	Observational study using survey data from before and after Denmark's 1998 ban	Daily gain in weaner pigs	2.6% decrease (effect of discon-tinuing use)
Liu, Miller, and McNamara, 2005	2000	Observational study using survey data	Average daily gain	Maximum effect of approximately 2.9% (effect of use)[d]
			Variability	Maximum effect of a decrease of 28.4% (effect of use)[e]
			Profits	$1,670 loss in profits for typical farm (effect of discontinuing use)[f]
McBride, Key, and Mathews, 2008	2004 data	Observational study using survey data	Total factor productivity of finishing hog production	No statistically significant effect (effect of use)
			Total factor productivity of nursery pigs	Large statistically significant positive effect (effect of use)
Hogberg, Raper, and Oehmke, 2009	Effect sizes of production purpose antibiotic use discontinuation from 1950-1985	Modeled production functions	Total costs	Vary by producer type and by cost-level of user

Source	Time of study	Type of study	Outcome	Effect size of production-purpose antibiotic use or discontinuation
Oliver and Wells, 2013	2013	Experimental study comparing controls, antibiotics, and an antibiotic alternative	Total costs	Vary by producer type and by cost-level of user
			Average daily growth of nursery pigs	8.8% increase (effect of use)
Nemechek et al., 2013	2013	Experimental study comparing controls, antibiotics, and an antibiotic alternative	Average daily growth of nursery pigs	5.4% (effect of use)
			Growth per unit of feed in nursery pigs	3.3% increase (effect of use)
Key and McBride, 2014	2009 data	Observational study using survey data	Productivity of finishing hog facilities	1.0% increase, but not statistically significant (effect of use)
			Annual variation in production	1.4% decrease, but not statistically significant (effect of use)

[a] Percentage calculated from averages reported in Table 11 of Cromwell, 2002.

[b] Brorsen et al. (2002) report values of $0.46 and $2.76. These were updated to 2013 dollars using the Consumer Price Index (CPI).

[c] Miller et al. (2003) report a value of $0.59. This was updated to 2013 dollars using the CPI.

[d] This is the effect of use of feeding antibiotics as growth promoters to pigs for 75 days; the largest effects were found at 75 days. The percentage was calculated using numbers in Table 5 of Liu, Miller, and McNamara, 2005.

[e] This is the effect of use of feeding antibiotics as growth promoters to pigs for 65 days; the largest effects were found at 65 days. The percentage was calculated using numbers in Table 5 of Liu, Miller, and McNamara, 2005.

[f] Liu, Miller, and McNamara (2005) report a value of $1,400. This was updated to 2013 dollars using the CPI. Source: Compiled by USDA, Economic Research Service from literature survey.

Brorsen et al. (2002) summarize scientific studies from the later 1980s and the 1990s of the effects of specific antibiotics on feed efficiency, mortality, and sort loss (of animals falling outside the packer-specified weight range) in hogs. They find improvements in the "feed-to-gain" ratio from subtherapeutic levels of antibiotics fed to grower/finisher hogs between -1 percent (a decline) to 5 percent. The mean improvement was 2.74 percent. After reviewing two studies, Brorsen and coauthors note a mean level of mortality reduction of 0.75 percentage points; however, in one of the two studies, feeding subtherapeutic antibiotics had no statistically significant effect on finisher pig mortality. Summarizing three studies, Brorsen and coauthors find that sort losses at slaughter were reduced by $0.60 per pig by using antibiotic growth promotants (value updated from $0.46 to 2013 dollars using the CPI). The authors then use their findings in a simulation to find that producers benefit by $3.60 (2013$) per pig from using subtherapeutic antibiotics.

More recent experimental research shows much smaller effects or no effects of antimicrobials added to feed. Dritz and coauthors (2002) conducted a controlled trial of 24,099 pigs at three multisite production systems. They compared growth rate and feed efficiency of nursery and finishing hogs according to administration of antimicrobials in feed. The researchers found that growth rate of nursery pigs fed antimicrobials improved by a statistically significant 5 percent. However, growth rate of finishing pigs and feed efficiency of finishing pigs and nursery pigs were not improved by the use of antimicrobials in feed.

Turning to farm-level analyses using survey data, Miller and coauthors (2005) use 1990 and 1995 swine surveys by the National Animal Health Monitoring Systems (NAHMS) to analyze the association between growth-promoting antibiotics and outcomes at grower/finisher operations. They are specifically interested in average daily gain, the average number of pounds of feed fed for each pound gained (feed conversion ratio), and the mortality rate over the prior 6 months. One issue with comparing farms that use growth-promoting antibiotics with those that do not is that the farm types may differ in other significant ways that could affect the outcomes. The authors therefore control for some of these relevant features by performing regression analysis in which they estimate the effects of antibiotic use on outcomes, controlling for region, size of operation, the year of the survey, the number of days in the growth phase, whether the producer was independent or under contract, and if the building had no outside access. They found that the more days that antibiotics were fed, the greater the improvements in average daily gain and the feed conversion ratio. Antibiotics fed over a longer time were also associated with a lowered mortality rate. For a representative grower/finisher operation, antibiotics were predicted to improve average daily gain by 0.5 percent and the feed conversion ratio by 1.1 percent. They were also predicted to reduce mortality by 0.22 percentage points.

Liu, Miller, and McNamara (2005) use updated 2000 NAHMS data to examine many of the same measures as Miller and coauthors (2003). Like the 2003 study using earlier versions of NAHMS, Liu et al. found the longer that growth-promoting antibiotics were fed, the greater the average daily gain. Liu and coauthors examine the effect of the number of days of feeding growth-promoting antibiotics on the average daily gain and the variability of hog weight and find that feeding growth-promoting antibiotics for 2 to 3 months increases weight and decreases variability. Variability in size and weight is an important factor in farm profitability risk; hogs outside a specified range may incur price penalties at market.

Turning to the research on effects before and after countrywide bans, antimicrobial growth-promoters were phased out from Danish pork production beginning in 1998, with a full voluntary ban on antimicrobials for growth promotion in weaner pigs by 2000. In a study of 150 farrow-to- finish operations, researchers examined post-weaning diarrhea occurrence requiring antibiotic treatment in the 6 months before and after the ban (WHO, 2002, p. 32, citing Larsen, 2002). The number of treatments increased from 0.4 per pig-month in the 6 months prior to the ban to approximately 1.0 treatments per pig-month in the 6 months after the ban (WHO, 2002, p. 33). The same study also showed that the incidence of diarrhea treatment of finisher pigs increased after the ban, but returned to pre-ban levels within 1 year (WHO, 2002, p. 33). Comparing the daily gain in weaner pigs in the 3 years prior to the ban (1995-1998) to the 3 years after (1999-2001) shows a 2.6-percent decrease from 422gm/day (1995-1998) to 411gm/day (1999-2001) (Dibner and Richards, 2005, citing Callesen, 2003).

Also examining the Danish ban, Kjeldsen (2002), comparing 62 Danish finisher herds in periods before and after 1998, reported that only a fraction (11 percent) of herds experienced 'permanent' problems such as reduced daily gain or increased diarrhea treatments. Kjeldsen does not report standard errors, so it is not possible to know whether changes were statistically significant. For finisher hogs in the post-ban period, the increase in daily gain was not as great as before the ban; daily gain did not decline, but rather did not grow as quickly as previously. This effect seems to be eliminated over time. However, the mortality rate of finisher hogs did increase marginally in the post-ban period (from 3.2 percent in 1997-1998 to 3.4 percent in 1998-1999). Kjeldsen notes that weaner pigs did not fare as well as their adult counterparts. Weaner pigs saw a 5-percent decline in daily gain in the initial post-ban period, a 0.7-percent point increase in mortality, and a 3-percent increase in the length of time it took to reach 30kg.

Robertsson and Lendeheim (1994) describe the effects of Sweden's 1986 ban on antimicrobial growth promoters on piglet health and hog production. They find that after the ban, post-weaning piglet mortality increased significantly, and the time to reach 25kg also increased. Hayes and coauthors (1999) report that overall, the effects of the Swedish ban on operations with good hygiene practices were minimal, and they note that many farmers converted to a form of all-in, all-out production to reduce hygiene issues.

FARM-LEVEL PRODUCTIVITY EFFECTS OF PRODUCTION-PURPOSE ANTIBIOTIC USE: HOGS

To examine farm-level productivity changes attributable to production-purpose antibiotics, researchers compare the net income from livestock of farms that use production-purpose antibiotics to those that do not. After controlling for potential confounders, Miller and coauthors (2003) first estimate the effects of growth-promoting antibiotics on average daily gain, feed efficiency, and the mortality rate in grower/finisher operations (results described above). To predict the economic impact of these effects, they use their estimates combined with other economic values in a "swine enterprise budgeting model" that they do not specify. They report that growth-promoting antibiotics increased profits by $0.75 per pig marketed (2013$). This amounts to a growth-promoting antibiotic contribution of 9 percent of the net returns of typical Midwestern grow-finish operations. Note that these economic outcomes also assume that there would be no market-level effects of widespread changes in antimicrobial growth-promoters.

Economic effects of production-purpose antibiotic use extend not just to direct effects on productivity of animals and the associated increased revenue if production-purpose antibiotics are less costly than the benefits. Production-purpose antibiotics may also be used to increase uniformity among animals, as noted above. As shown by Liu, Miller, and McNamara (2005; described above), growth-promoting antibiotics can decrease the variability in hog weight in grower/finisher operations. The researchers employ their estimated effects of growth-promoting antibiotic use on average daily gain and variability to predict effects of growth-promoting antibiotic withdrawal on a typical hog farm. They find that removal of growth-promoting antibiotics would lead to a $1,670 loss in profits for an individual operation due to changes in variation in pig liveweight (2013$). The authors assume that no other market changes occurred with the removal of growth-promoting antibiotics, which would not be the case if a policy were adopted banning use of all production-purpose antibiotics for all producers.

An issue with comparing farms that use production-purpose antibiotics with those that do not is that farms may use production-purpose antibiotics because they have poor outcomes due to other factors. Hence, the relationship between production-purpose antibiotic use and outcomes may reflect the effect of the poor outcomes on the use of production-purpose antibiotics, rather than the effect of the production-purpose antibiotics on the outcomes. If this is the case, cross-sectional analyses may underestimate the effect of production-purpose antibiotics on outcomes. To address this potential estimation problem, McBride, Key, and Mathews (2008) employ a sample-selection model applied to 2004 ARMS survey data of U.S. hog producers. They first estimate the likelihood that a farm will use antibiotics for growth promotion, and then controlling for this likelihood, they estimate the effects of growth-promoting antibiotics on total factor productivity using a production frontier approach. Total factor productivity is an economic term that refers to the efficiency with which inputs are used. The authors measure total factor productivity using an index defined as total output (weight gain) divided by total expenditures on inputs. They find that antibiotics as growth promoters have no significant effects on the total factor productivity of finisher-hog production. However, they find that growth-promoting antibiotics result in a substantial increase in the productivity for operations specializing in nursery pigs.

Key and McBride (2014) update the earlier work using the 2009 ARMS data for finishing operations. The authors use data to estimate a production frontier model, which describes the greatest amount of output that can be produced at each level of inputs (the "frontier"). To test whether antibiotics provided for growth promotion allow producers to use inputs more or less efficiently, the authors estimate whether growth-promoting antibiotic use is correlated with being closer or further away from the frontier. They first "match" each farm using antibiotics as growth promoters to a similar farm not using antibiotics for growth promotion. In this way, the authors create two groups that are as similar as possible across observable factors that may affect outcomes, thereby removing potential confounding effects of factors that may

Appendix Table A3. Summary of literature on effects of production-purpose antibiotic use and discontinuation on animal- and farm-level outcomes in beef and dairy cattle

Source	Time of studies summarized	Type of study	Outcome	Effect size of production purpose antibiotic use
Gilliam and Martin, 1975	Studies from 1960 to 1969	Summary of prior research	Average daily gain, beef cattle	6%[a]
			Feed/gain, beef cattle	7%[a]
			Average daily gain, veal calves	19%[a]
			Gain/feed, veal calves	-9%[a]
CAST, 1981	1950s	Review of experimental studies	Weight gain	5% (beef)
			Growth	12% to 60% (dairy calves)
Mathews, 2002	Study from 1987	Summary of prior research	Feed efficiency	4%
			Growth rate	6%
Lawrence and Ibarburu, 2007	Studies published in 1989	Review of literature	Average daily gain, stocker cattle	-21% to 11%; average simulated effect of 6.87%
	Studies published in 1991 and 2000	Review of literature	Average daily gain, feedlot cattle	-9% to 11%; average simulated effect of 3.37%
	Studies published in 1984 and 1995	Review of literature	Feed/gain, feedlot cattle	-8% to 19%; average simulated effect of -2.69%
		Estimated effects using farm-level cost-of-production budget model	Production costs, stocker operations	$11.06/head (effect of discontinuing use; 2013$)[b]
			Production costs, beef feedlots	$6.77/head (effect of discontinuing use; 2013$)[c]

[a] Calculated from values in Table 1, Gilliam and Martin (1975).

[b] Lawrence and Ibarburu (2007) report costs of $9.57 in 2006 dollars. This was updated to 2013 dollars using the CPI-U.

[c] Lawrence and Ibarburu (2007) report costs of $5.86 in 2006 dollars. This was updated to 2013 dollars using the CPI-U.

Source: Compiled by USDA, Economic Research Service from literature survey.

be correlated with antibiotic use. They find that growth-promoting antibiotics improve productivity by about 1.0 percent, but this result is not statistically different from zero. Key and McBride also find that growth-promoting antibiotic use is associated with a reduced annual variation in production, although again the result is not statistically significantly different from zero.

Hogberg, Raper, and Oehmke (2009) develop models of differently sized farms to evaluate how a ban on antibiotics for growth promotion would impact hog producers. They are particularly concerned with the fact that growth-promoting antibiotics may allow for economies of scale in hog production. They argue that growth-promoting antibiotic use has been important in generating the current U.S. industry structure of highly concentrated production. Their analysis uses estimated effects of removal of antibiotics from an unpublished dataset described in Cromwell (2002). Again, no estimates of statistical significance are reported in Cromwell, so it is difficult to ascertain whether these effects are precise or even statistically different from zero. Cromwell reports that removal of production-purpose antibiotics would lead to a 9.6-percent decrease in litters per sow per year, an 8.8-percent decrease in the survival rate of piglets, and a 13.3-percent decrease in average daily gain, as well as a number of attendant changes. Hogberg et al. apply these changes to data on other herds to predict the effects of removing growth-promoting antibiotics. For example, they multiply the percent change in feed efficiency due to growth-promoting antibiotic removal by the amount of feed to calculate a change in the total amount of feed used. Implicit in Hogberg et al.'s assumption is that producers feed the same number of hogs to market weight. They assume that producers do not make changes to production practices aside from increasing labor in response to removal of antibiotics. Finally, Hogberg and coauthors assume that prices for meat do not change after the ban. These problematic aspects of the study should be kept in mind when interpreting results. Hogberg et al. find that a full ban on antibiotics as growth promoters would be unprofitable for many producers, with the largest effects among small producers. The ban would also increase labor costs, as employees require more education to diagnose and monitor hogs for disease. Hogberg and coauthors predict that economies of scale in breed-to-wean operations would be reduced.

Animal-Level Effects of Production-Purpose Antibiotic Use – Beef and Dairy

The productivity effects of production-purpose antibiotics in beef cattle are mixed; see Table A3. The CAST (1981) study reported that experiments in the 1950s showed an increase in weight gain among beef cattle from production-purpose antibiotics of 5 percent. Summarizing literature, Lawrence and Ibarburu (2007) report that production-purpose antibiotic use in stocker cattle altered average daily gain in the range of decreasing it by 21 percent or increasing it by 27 percent. Studies on feedlot cattle show a range of a decrease of 9 percent to an increase of 11 percent in average daily gain. Lawrence and Ibarburu also note that production-purpose antibiotic effects on weight gain per unit of feed range from an increase of 19 percent to a decline of 8 percent. The authors use the data from several experiments to simulate a distribution of effects of production-purpose antibiotics. They estimate an average effect of 6.87 percent on daily growth among stocker cattle and a 3.37-percent increase for beef feedlots. They also estimate that antimicrobial therapy is associated with a 2.69- percent decrease in the amount of feed per unit of weight gain.

Mathews (2002) also summarizes prior studies and notes improvements in feed efficiency and growth rates ranging from no effect to 8 percent. For later analysis, Mathews assumes a growth rate effect of 6 percent and a feed efficiency effect of 4 percent.

In a 1975 report, Gilliam and Martin summarize research that is largely from the 1960s. In their economic analysis, they assume an effect on average daily weight gain in beef cattle of about 6 percent from using antibiotics in feed (from 2.166 pounds without production-purpose antibiotics to 2.292 with production-purpose antibiotics), and approximately 7 percent more feed required per unit of weight gain (about 7 percent slower gain). For veal calves, Gilliam and Martin assume an increased weight gain per day from production-purpose antibiotics of about 19 percent and a 9-percent decline in the weight gain per unit of feed.

Dairy calves have also been shown to have faster growth rates from production-purpose antibiotic use in experimental research. Summarizing studies from the 1950s, CAST (1981) reports that different types of antibiotics had effects on dairy calf growth of between 12 and 60 percent.

Farm-Level Effects of Production-Purpose Antibiotics – Beef

There has been little research into the farm-level effects of production-purpose antibiotic use or discontinuation among beef producers. Using the estimates of productivity impacts reported above, Lawrence and Ibarburu (2006) model the effects that stopping use of production-purpose antibiotics would have on production costs employing a farm-level cost-of-production model. They find that forgoing 'antimicrobial therapy' would increase production costs by $11.06 per head in stocker operations and $6.77 per head in beef feedlots (2013$).

Market-Level Effects of Production-Purpose Antibiotics on Supply and Price

Researchers have used the effect sizes found in the research reviewed above to estimate the impacts a ban on production-purpose antibiotics would have in the United States. In this type of study, researchers employ models of the industry and parameters from what happened after similar bans to predict what may happen from a U.S. ban. Many of these analyses were done when the United States first started contemplating restrictions on production-purpose antibiotic use in the 1970s. Later research appears correlated with more recent policy proposals to restrict use.

In an early analysis, Allan and Burbee (1972) examined the effects of a ban on subtherapeutic antibiotic use on production, costs, and prices of broilers and turkeys. They analyzed several scenarios, including ones in which producers generate the same level of output and others in which producers maintain existing lengths of feeding time (and produce less). Assuming that subtherapeutic use increases feed efficiency, to generate the same level of output producers must feed birds for longer or feed more birds for the same length of time. Allan and Burbee find an assortment of effects, ranging from producers reducing to increasing costs and from prices increasing a few cents to several dollars (see Table A4).

Gilliam and Martin (1975) use partial budgeting and parameters on effects of antimicrobial feed additives from experimental research from the 1960s to estimate the effect on total costs and prices of a ban on use of antimicrobial feed additives in hogs. They make several strong assumptions, including that producers will not alter any behavior in response to the ban and that

Appendix Table A2. Summary of literature on effects of production-purpose antibiotic use and discontinuation on animal- and farm-level outcomes in hogs

Source	Time of study	Type of study	Outcome	Effect size of production-purpose antibiotic use or discontinuation
Cromwell, 1991	1950-1985	Summary of experimental studies	Daily gain, young pigs	16.4% (effect of use)
			Feed/gain, young pigs	-6.9% (effect of use)
			Daily gain, growing phase	10.6% (effect of use)
			Feed/gain, growing phase	-4.5% (effect of use)
			Daily gain, grower/finisher pigs	4.2% (effect of use)
			Feed/gain, young pigs	-2.2% (effect of use)
Robertsson and Lend-eheim, 1994	Before and after 1986	Observational study surveying a set of farms before and after Sweden's 1986 ban	Post-weaning piglet mortality	0.4-0.5 percentage point increase (effect of discontinuing use)
			Number of pigs weaned/litter	4.9% (effect of use)[a]
			Percentage piglets surviving until weaning	1.7 percentage points (effect of use)[a]
			Percentage of breeding pigs that farrowed	7 percentage points (effect of use)
Cromwell, 2002	Studies largely from the 1960s	Summary of experimental studies	Live pigs born per litter	3.0% (effect of use)[a]
			Number of pigs weaned/litter	4.9% (effect of use)[a]
			Percentage piglets surviving until weaning	1.7 percentage points (effect of use)[a]
			Percentage of breeding pigs that farrowed	7 percentage points (effect of use)
Dritz, Tokach, Goodband, and Nelssen, 2002	Before 2002	Experimental study	Growth rate, nursery pigs	5% (effect of use)
			Growth rate, finishing pigs	No statistically significant effect (effect of use)

Source	Time of study	Type of study	Outcome	Effect size of production-purpose antibiotic use or discontinuation
			Feed efficiency, nursery pigs and finishing pigs	No statistically significant effect (effect of use)
Brorsen et al., 2002	Studies from 1980s and 1990s	Summaries of scientific studies	Feed efficiency, finishing pigs	-1% to 5% (effect of use), average of 2.74%
			Mortality reduction, finishing pigs	0.75 percentage points
			Sort loss reduction	\$0.60/hog (effect of use)[b]
	Simulation	Benefit per hog	\$3.59/hog (effect of use)[b]	
World Health Organization (WHO), 2002 citing Larsen, 2002	Before and after 1998	Observational study using data from before and after	Number of antibiotic treatments	Increased from 0.4 per pig-month to 1.0 per pig-month (effect of discontinuing use)
			Incidence of diarrhea treatment in finisher hogs	Initial increase but return to pre-ban levels within 1 year (effect of discontinuing use)
Kjeldsen, 2002	Before and after 1998	Observational study using survey data from before and after Sweden's national ban	'Permanent' problems like reduced daily gain or increased diarrhea treatments	11% of herds showed problems (effect of discontinuing use)
			Mortality rate of finisher hogs	0.2 percentage point increase (effect of discontinuing use)
			Daily gain of weaner pigs	5% decline (effect of discontinuing use)
			Mortality of weaner pigs	0.7 percentage point increase (effect of discontinuing use)
			Length of time for weaner pigs to reach 30kg	3% increase (effect of discontinuing use)

Appendix Table A2. (Continued)

Source	Time of study	Type of study	Outcome	Effect size of production-purpose antibiotic use or discontinuation
Miller et al., 2003	1990 and 1995	Observational study using survey data	Average daily gain	0.5% (effect of use)
			Feed conversion ratio	1.1% (effect of use)
			Profits	$0.75 per pig marketed (effect of use)[c]
			Mortality rate	-0.22 percentage points (effect of use)
Dibner and Richards, 2005, citing Callesen, 2003	1995-1998 and 1999-2001	Observational study using survey data from before and after Denmark's 1998 ban	Daily gain in weaner pigs	2.6% decrease (effect of discontinuing use)
Liu, Miller, and McNamara, 2005	2000	Observational study using survey data	Average daily gain	Maximum effect of approximately 2.9% (effect of use)[d]
			Variability	Maximum effect of a decrease of 28.4% (effect of use)[e]
			Profits	$1,670 loss in profits for typical farm (effect of discontinuing use)[f]
McBride, Key, and Mathews, 2008	2004 data	Observational study using survey data	Total factor productivity of finishing hog production	No statistically significant effect (effect of use)
			Total factor productivity of nursery pigs	Large statistically significant positive effect (effect of use)
Hogberg, Raper, and Oehmke, 2009	Effect sizes of production purpose antibiotic use discontinuation from 1950-1985	Modeled production functions	Total costs	Vary by producer type and by cost-level of user

Source	Time of study	Type of study	Outcome	Effect size of production-purpose antibiotic use or discontinuation
Oliver and Wells, 2013	2013	Experimental study comparing controls, antibiotics, and an antibiotic alternative	Total costs	Vary by producer type and by cost-level of user
			Average daily growth of nursery pigs	8.8% increase (effect of use)
Nemechek et al., 2013	2013	Experimental study comparing controls, antibiotics, and an antibiotic alternative	Average daily growth of nursery pigs	5.4% (effect of use)
			Growth per unit of feed in nursery pigs	3.3% increase (effect of use)
Key and McBride, 2014	2009 data	Observational study using survey data	Productivity of finishing hog facilities	1.0% increase, but not statistically significant (effect of use)
			Annual variation in production	1.4% decrease, but not statistically significant (effect of use)

[a] Percentage calculated from averages reported in Table 11 of Cromwell, 2002.

[b] Brorsen et al. (2002) report values of $0.46 and $2.76. These were updated to 2013 dollars using the Consumer Price Index (CPI).

[c] Miller et al. (2003) report a value of $0.59. This was updated to 2013 dollars using the CPI.

[d] This is the effect of use of feeding antibiotics as growth promoters to pigs for 75 days; the largest effects were found at 75 days. The percentage was calculated using numbers in Table 5 of Liu, Miller, and McNamara, 2005.

[e] This is the effect of use of feeding antibiotics as growth promoters to pigs for 65 days; the largest effects were found at 65 days. The percentage was calculated using numbers in Table 5 of Liu, Miller, and McNamara, 2005.

[f] Liu, Miller, and McNamara (2005) report a value of $1,400. This was updated to 2013 dollars using the CPI. Source: Compiled by USDA, Economic Research Service from literature survey.

consumers will demand the same amount of pork regardless of price (also known as perfectly inelastic demand). Assuming no change in the amount of pork produced, the authors estimate a $0.30/lb increase in the retail price of pork and a total market-wide increase in production costs of $2.8 billion (2013$). For beef, the authors examine two scenarios: The first assumes that there is no change in the amount of pork produced, and the second assumes that the amount of pork produced declines. Gilliam and Martin note that to generate the same amount of beef without antimicrobial feed additives would raise market-wide production costs by $1.4 billion and would increase retail price by about 8.9 cents per pound (2013 dollars). Assuming instead that the number of cattle placed on feed and the length of time on feed did not change, Gilliam and Martin estimate that beef production would fall by under 2 percent without antimicrobial feed additives, with an attendant 9.9-percent increase in price.

In another early study, Dworkin (1976) analyzes the effects on costs, production, revenues, and retail prices of a ban on subtherapeutic use of tetracyclines in feedlot cattle and swine under four different scenarios. These scenarios depend on whether producers use an alternative feed additive to maintain growth levels lowered by discontinuing subtherapeutic antibiotics and whether producers feed animals for the same length of time (thereby producing less meat) or for longer to produce the same amount. The model used is not stated and is therefore not possible to evaluate, but it assumes that there is no supply response to a change in antibiotic use. Under a scenario where animals are not fed an alternative medicated feed and are fed for the same length of time as before a ban, Dworkin finds that costs per head actually decline while market prices increase—as production declines, revenues increase.

Mann and Paulsen (1976) use a 42-equation simulation model to estimate the effect of a ban on anti- microbial feed additives in both the short and the long term. They examine effects not only for hogs, but also for cattle and poultry. Their model incorporates parameters and relationships indicative of the time period (pre-1975). They find that prices would rise permanently under a ban and that pork producers would experience the greatest impact. In the first 3 years of the ban, prices would rise a great deal but then fall again (although not to pre-ban levels). For pork, prices in the short term would rise by as much as 4.5 percent over predicted prices without a ban. They note that despite this increase, the average hog producer would be unlikely to experience "financial disaster" from the ban. They find that quantity produced would decline but that prices would increase more than proportionately, leading to profits in the short term. Beef, broilers, and turkeys would also experience price increases in the early stages of a ban (1.1 percent for beef, 2.2 percent for broilers, and 3.4 percent for turkeys). Again, these price increases would be mitigated in later stages of the ban.

The USDA (1978) uses an econometric simulation that incorporates all livestock sectors to predict the effects of different forms of a ban on selected animal drugs fed at subtherapeutic levels. The simulation is based on estimates taken from the experimental literature and from experts on the effects of antimicrobial use on the productivity of animals; the authors note that these estimates are from the 1950s and 1960s and show wide variance. Another crucial assumption of the methodology is that producers make no changes to mitigate the effects of discontinuing subtherapeutic antibiotic use. Using their model that incorporates predictions from the hog, broiler, cattle, and turkey industries, the USDA researchers estimate changes in price, quantity, and farm incomes for 1 to 5 years after a ban. The largest effects occur in the first year of the ban, after which variables adjust closer to pre-ban levels. The poultry sector sees the largest effects on prices and quantities; under an assumption of "moderate efficiency" of subtherapeutic antibiotics, broiler price increases by 13 percent in the first year after the ban. By year 5, this has lowered to 2.25 percent. Hog prices are predicted to rise by 5.02 percent in the first year and 1.14 percent by year 5. For fed beef, the changes are the smallest; price increases by just 1.68 percent in the first year, declining to no-effect by year 5.

Quantity effects in the USDA report follow a similar trajectory to prices. Again, the largest effect is in the amount of broilers produced; this is predicted to decline by 8.24 percent in the first year. By year 5, the broiler effect is predicted to be reduced to 2.16 percent. Corresponding year 1 and year 5 numbers for hogs are a 4.86-percent decline and a 0.84-percent decline. The amount of fed beef produced is predicted to slightly increase. The USDA report also finds that cash receipts for livestock products are predicted to increase for all livestock types in the first year after the ban. The receipts remain positive for 5 years after the ban for all species except hogs, which show a 0.2 percent decline.

A final note about the USDA study is that it also explores the effects on the grain sector of a ban on use of subtherapeutic antibiotics. Operating under the assumption that livestock producers will require more feed due to lowered feed efficiency, the USDA researchers also estimate the effects on prices and quantities of feed crops. They find a decline in prices and cash receipts for feed crops.

Wade and Barkley (1992) perform static equilibrium analysis to estimate the change in prices and quantity of a ban on subtherapeutic antibiotic use in pork. They first econometrically estimate the supply and demand equations for pork using data from 1959 to 1989. Wade and Barkley then assume that a ban on subtherapeutic use in pork would decrease the supply of pork by 4 percent. They argue that consumers would be willing to pay more for meat perceived to be safer and therefore assume that demand for pork would increase by 5 percent under a ban. This leads to a 3.2-percent increase in price and a 2.8-percent decrease in quantity produced. Note that these authors look only at the pork sector; the ban is assumed to only affect hogs, not chicken or beef.

Hayes and coauthors (1999 and 2001) employ a quarterly simulation model of the U.S. livestock industry to estimate what would happen if the United States banned over-the-counter antibiotics in hog production (but not in poultry or beef). In the model, market equilibrium price and quantity for pork, beef, and chicken are jointly determined. Hayes and coauthors use estimates from the Swedish experience to characterize impacts on average daily growth, feed conversion, and mortality rates of both nursery pigs and hogs at grower/finisher operations. In their 'most likely' scenario, Hayes et al. suggest that a ban would reduce average daily growth of smaller pigs by 1.3 percent, and by 1.8 percent for larger pigs. They assume that the feed conversion rate would decline by 1.7 percent for the smaller pigs and 1.5 percent for the larger pigs. Finally, they use expected changes in mortality rates of 1.5 percent for smaller pigs and 0.04 percent for larger pigs. These estimates arise from historical analyses of how Sweden's ban impacted the Swedish hog industry and take into account producer changes in practices in reaction to the ban. Hayes and coauthors feed these estimates into a model to estimate effects of a possible U.S. ban on production costs and profits. They factor in adjustment costs that producers incur to blunt the impact of not using over-the-counter antibiotics, such as additional space for nursery and finishing periods. They conclude that in their 'most likely' scenario production costs would increase by $8.46 per head in the first year of the ban and would decline over 10 years (2013$). Profits would decline by $5.83 per head initially, eventually reaching a loss of only $1.10 per head after 10 years (2013$).

The National Research Council (1999) performs a very simplistic analysis to predict the effects of a ban on per capita costs. Based on suggestions largely from a handful of experts (not experimental studies or other research), the NRC combines predictions of the changes in feed efficiency with current prices and quantities to estimate changes in per capita costs. The NRC

Appendix Table A5. Comparison of consumer and producer surplus measures from prior research on market-level effects of restrictions on production-purpose antibiotic use in livestock production

Study	Year study was published	Livestock types included	Aggregate costs per year (million dollars)[f]
Allen and Burbee; Gilliam et al.[a]			
Losses to consumers	1972; 1973	Beef, pork, broilers, and turkeys	18,161
Dworkin[a]			
Losses to consumers	1976	Beef and pork only	6,866
Mann and Paulsen[a]			
Losses to consumers	1976	Beef, pork, broilers, and turkeys	1,861
Headly[a]			
Losses to consumers, Scenario I[b]	1978	Beef, pork,	3,979
Losses to consumers, Scenario II[c]		broilers, and turkeys	4,621 15,016
U.S. Dept. of Agriculture[a]			
Losses to consumers, Scenario II[d]	1978	Beef, pork, broilers, and turkeys	
Wade and Barkley			
Losses to consumers	1992	Pork only	24
Losses to producers			26
National Research Council/Institute of Medicine			
Extra amount spent on meat by U.S. population; ban with substitutes	1998	Beef, pork, broilers, and turkeys	1,826
Extra amount spent on meat by U.S. population; ban without substitutes			3,667
Hayes et al.			
Losses to consumers	1999	Pork only	1,069
Losses to producers			229

Mathews			
Losses to consumers; full ban	2002	Beef only	810
Losses to consumers; partial ban			123
Brorsen et al.			
Losses to consumers; full ban[e]	2002	Beef, pork, and poultry	216
Losses to producers; full ban[e]			100

[a] Data from Table 45 of Council for Agricultural Science and Technology (CAST), 1981; 5-year totals divided by 5 to give annual amounts.

[b] Ban penicillin and tetracycline.

[d] Moderate efficiency; ban penicillin, tetracyclines, sulfa drugs, and nitrofurans.

[e] Elasticities of farm supply for beef, pork, and poultry are 0.5. fNumbers adjusted to 2013 dollars using the Consumer Price Index.

Source: Table developed from Mathews (2001).

assumes no changes in prices or quantities due to changes in subtherapeutic antibiotic use, basically ignoring economic theory. The researchers find price changes of between 2 and 8 cents per pound (2013$), which translates into extra costs each year for a family of four of $0.48 and $1.05 (2013$).

Brorsen and coauthors (2002) perform a straightforward market analysis of the effects of a ban on subtherapeutic antibiotic use on consumer and producer surplus. They examine the effects in both the short and long runs and find consumer surplus losses ranging from $144 to $262 million (2013$) and producer surplus losses ranging from $53 to $172 million (2013$).

Mathews (2002) models the beef sector to estimate the economic effects of a reduction in antibiotic use. Mathews used a least-cost feeding model to simulate and compare total annual liveweight of fed-cattle production with no ban, a partial ban, and a full ban of low-level antimicrobial drug use in feeding cattle. Using a growth rate effect of 6 percent, and a feed efficiency effect of 4 percent, Mathews estimates that a full ban on low-level antimicrobial drug use would be associated with feeding animals for a longer period, as average daily gain is assumed to be lower. He finds that animals would be fed for 8.4 percent longer but would still reach final weights 1.4 percent lower. This would result in a 9-percent decrease in total production. Further, cattle prices would increase by $3.41 per hundredweight (2013$ dollars; approximately 3 percent).

The various market-level studies also generally report changes from the reduction of production-purpose antibiotics to consumer and/or producer surplus. Consumer surplus, a measure of satisfaction that people receive from consuming goods, is defined as the difference between the amount that consumers would be willing and able to pay for a good and what they actually pay. Similarly, producer surplus is defined as the difference between the amount that a producer of a good receives and the minimum amount that he or she would be willing to accept for the good. Appendix B describes calculation of consumer and producer surplus in more detail. Table A5 shows market-level study estimates of changes in consumer and producer surplus (and in one case the extra amount that consumers would need to pay to purchase the same quantity of meat). The estimated costs to consumers (the change in consumer surplus) range from $24 million per year to over $1 billion.

Demand Effects of Production-Purpose Antibiotic Use or Discontinuation

Little research examines the willingness of consumers to pay more for meat that has not been raised with production-purpose antibiotics. Lusk and coauthors (2006) conducted an experiment on shoppers' willingness to pay for antibiotic-free pork and found that people were willing to pay a 76.7 percent premium, with a price premium of between $0.68 and $4.72 (updated to 2013$). Providing shoppers with information on antibiotics did not influence preferences. Bernard, Pan, and Sirolli (2005) surveyed Delaware residents regarding product attributes of chicken and found that about 80 percent of respondents favored labeling chickens that were treated with antibiotics.

Appendix B: Market Model Description and Further Results

Model Description

To generate estimates of the effects of a ban on production-purpose antibiotic use on market-level outcomes, we develop a simple supply and demand model.

As described in Figure B1, the reduction in production caused by a ban on antibiotics is shown as a shift in the supply curve from Supply to Supply'. At the initial price, the shift causes the supply to contract from Q_0 to Q_1. Assume the antibiotic ban changes output among production-purpose antibiotic users by $X\%$, holding all else constant, including prices. Let $J\%$ be the proportion of production that uses production-purpose antibiotics. For notational simplicity, define the output reduction factor:

$$A = (100 + (X\% \times J\%))/100, \text{ so } Q_1 = AQ_0.$$

The elasticity of both supply curves is given as $E_S = \frac{\%\Delta Q_s}{\%\Delta P_s}$ and the elasticity of the demand curve $E_D = \frac{\%\Delta Q_D}{\%\Delta P_D}$.

Given the supply and demand elasticities E_S and E_D, the reduction factor A, and initial output Q_0, we can derive the new equilibrium after the ban.

To compute the equilibrium quantity Q_2 we use the fact that the increase in price (from P_0 to P_2) resulting from the move up the demand curve (from Q_0 to Q_2) must be the same as the increase in price resulting from the move up the supply curve Supply' from Q_1 to Q_2. Hence, the following condition must hold:

$$\%\Delta P_S = \%\Delta P_D \text{ or } \frac{\%\Delta Q_S}{E_S} = \frac{\%\Delta Q_D}{E_D} \text{ or } \frac{(Q_2 - Q_1)/Q_1}{E_S} = \frac{(Q_2 - Q_0)/Q_0}{E_D}.$$

Using the fact that $Q_1 = AQ_0$, we can solve for Q_2 :

$$Q_2 = AQ_0(E_D - E_S)/(E_D - AE_S).$$

Using Q_2, we can calculate P_2 from the movement up the demand curve from Q_0 to Q_2:

$$\%\Delta P_D = \%\Delta Q_D/E_D \text{ or } (P_2 - P_0)/P_0 = \frac{(Q_2 - Q_0)/Q_0}{E_D}$$

So: $$P_2 = P_0 \frac{(Q_2 - Q_0)/Q_0}{E_D} + P_0.$$

To assess the impacts of price and quantity changes on consumers and producers, economists use the concepts of consumer and producer surplus.

Consumer surplus is a measure of satisfaction that people receive from consuming goods and is defined as the difference between the amount that consumers would be willing and able to pay for a good and what they actually pay. Figure B1 mirrors Figure 10 in the main text, but with more notation. In Figure B1, consumer surplus for the original supply and demand curves is the area (a + b + c + d); most consumers would be willing to pay more for the product than the price that they did pay (P_0), and consumer surplus measures the difference between the market price and the demand curve. When production-purpose antibiotic use is restricted and the supply curve shifts to the left, consumer surplus is just the area (a); this reduction is due to the increased price paid by people still buying (area b + c) and the loss of surplus on the quantity that is no longer bought (area d). Hence we can see that in this scenario, restrictions on production-purpose antibiotic use would yield a loss in consumer surplus for consumers of broilers. Similarly, producer surplus is defined as the difference between the amount that a producer of a good receives and the minimum amount that he or she would be willing to accept for the good. In Figure B1, for the original supply and demand curves, the producer surplus is (e + f + g + h + I + j + k). After the supply curve shifts to the left, the producer surplus is (b + e + i); producers get added revenues from the higher price on what they are selling (area b + c), but at a higher cost (by c + f + g + k + j), and they are selling less, with a foregone producer surplus of (h) from the lost sales.

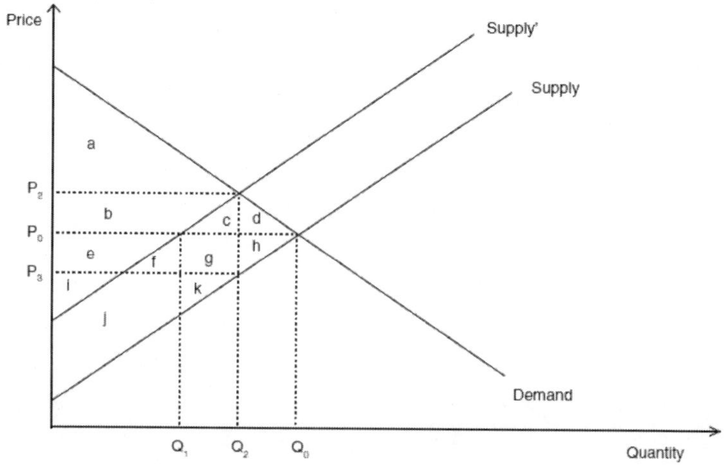

Source: USDA, Economic Research Service.

Appendix Figure B1. Supply and demand for meat.

Given Q_0, Q_1, Q_2, P_0, P_2, and P_3, we can, for small percentage changes *XX*, approximate the areas of the regions in the figure using simple geometry. The change in consumer surplus is the area b + c + d = $\frac{1}{2}(Q_2 + Q_0)(P_2 - P_0)$. The change in producer surplus is the area b-(f + g + h + j + k) = $\frac{1}{2}(Q_2 + Q_0)(P_3 - P_0)$.

We can calculate *PP3* as a movement down the supply curve from Q_0 to Q_2:

$$\%\Delta P_S = \%\Delta Q_S / E_S \text{ or } (P_3 - P_0)/P_0 = \frac{(Q_2 - Q_0)/Q_0}{E_S}$$

So: $P_3 = P_0 \frac{(Q_2 - Q_0)/Q_0}{E_S} + P_0$.

We can also estimate the changes in output and value of production for production using production-purpose antibiotics versus that not using antibiotic for such purposes. To do this, we assume that users and nonusers have the same elasticity of supply, but users produce *X%* more quantity at every price. Figure B2 shows that the supply curves of production-purpose antibiotic nonusers ($Supply_N$), production-purpose antibiotic users ($Supply_U$), and the market supply curves before (*Supply*) and after (*Supply'*) a ban. Prices are set at the market level, not at the individual-firm level; hence, only the market demand curve is shown.

The total market-level quantity is the sum of that produced by the users and the nonusers:

$$q_{N0} + q_{U0} = Q_0 \text{ and } q_{N2} + q_{U2} = Q_2,$$

Where $q_{N0} = \frac{(100 - J\%)}{100} Q_0$.

At the market level, when the supply curve shifts leftward, the shift elicits both a lower quantity produced and a higher price. Only the users experience a shift in their supply curve, so that it is equal to that of the nonusers. After the ban, users negotiate two competing forces: produce less as it is more expensive at every price to do so, and produce more as prices have risen. Thus, users' output shifts not to q_{N0}, but to q_{U2}.

Nonusers, on the other hand, experience no shift in their supply curve and only experience the market-level increase in price. Their production will increase, from q_{N0} to q_{U2}.

To calculate the changes in production by nonusers, we assume that nonusers and users have the same elasticity of supply (and likewise, that the market elasticity of supply is the same). To calculate their change in supply, we make use of the fact that $E_S = \frac{\%\Delta Q_S}{\%\Delta P_S}$, and we know the percentage change in price and the percentage of the starting production from nonusers:

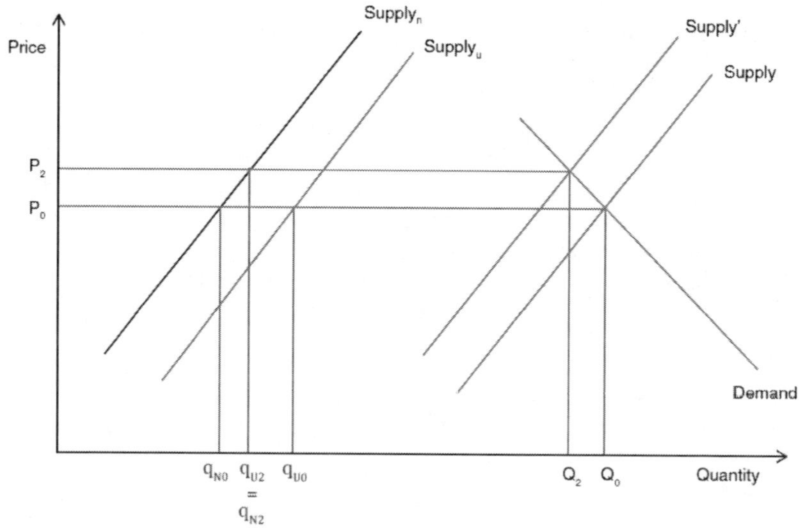

Source: USDA, Economic Research Service.

Appendix Figure B2. Supply and demand for meat, users versus nonusers of production-purpose antibiotics.

$$q_{N2} - q_{N0} = E_S\left(\frac{P_2 - P_0}{P_0}\right)\left(\frac{100 - \%J}{100}\right)Q_0$$

The change in production by users is therefore:

$Q_2 - Q_0 - (q_{N2} - q_{N0})$.

Since nonusers increase production, the amount that users decrease production is greater than the total market-level decrease in production.

The changes in the value of production for users and nonusers are calculated as:

$$q_{N2}\,P_2 - q_{N0}\,P_0 \quad \text{and} \quad q_{U2}\,P_2 - q_{U0}\,P_0.$$

Table B1. Consumer and producer surplus effects of full ban on production-purpose antibiotic use in hogs and broilers, Monte Carlo estimation results

	Scenario		
	1% - 3% reduction in supply from limiting production-purpose antibiotics		4% - 6% effect on young pig productivity from limiting production-purpose antibiotics
	Hogs	Broilers	Hogs
Consumer surplus (million $)	-263	-228	-110
	(101)	(102)	(35)
Producer surplus (million $)	-282	-183	-118
	(206)	(145)	(79)
Total surplus (million $)	-545	-411	-227
	(277)	(225)	(102)

Note: Dollar values are in 2012 dollars.
Source: USDA, Economic Research Service estimates.

Further Results

As described above, we calculate consumer and producer surplus using elasticities of supply and demand. Elasticities change along the points of a linear curve, and therefore our stated elasticities are only useful in evaluating small changes in price and quantity. To calculate percent changes in consumer and producer surplus would require extending the supply and demand curves toward zero prices, where the stated elasticities would no longer be valid.

In order to compare with earlier studies, we also calculate the changes in consumer and producer surplus (Table B1). As expected, these all decline. Consumers and producers equally share in the total surplus lost. Compared to prior studies, the effects on consumer surplus estimated here are either of the same order of magnitude, or, more often, smaller.

REFERENCES

Aarestrup, Frank M. (2003). "Effects of termination of AGP use on antimicrobials resistance in food animals." Page 6-11 in Working papers for the WHO international review panels evaluation. Document WHO/CDS/CPE/ZFK/2003.1a. World Health Organization, Geneva Switzerland.

Allen, G. & C. Burbee. (1972). *Economic consequences of the restricted use of antibiotics at subtherapeutic levels in broiler and turkey production.* Economic Research Service, U.S. Department of Agriculture. Farm Production Economics Division. November.

Bernard, J. C., Pan, X. & Sirolli, R. (2005). "Consumer attitude toward genetic modification and other possible production attributes for chicken," *Journal of Food Distribution Research*, *36*(2), 1-11.

Bhullar, K., Waglechner, N., Pawlowski, A., Koteva, K., Banks, E. D., Johnston, M. D., Barton, H. A. & Wright, G. D. (2012). "Antibiotic resistance is prevalent in an isolated cave microbiome." *PLoS ONE*, *7*(4), e34953.

Brorsen, B. W., T. Lehenbauer, D. Ji & J. Connor. (2002). "Economic impacts of banning subtherapeutic use of antibiotics in swine production," *Journal of Agricultural and Applied Economics*, *34(*3), 489-500.

Callesen, J. (2002). "Effects of termination of AGP-use on pig welfare and productivity," In: International Invitational Symposium; Beyond Antimicrobial Growth Promoters in Food Animal Production, November 6-7, 2002, Foulum, Denmark.

Chang, Q., W. Wang, R. Y., Gili, M. Lipstich. & W. P. Hanage. (2014). "Antibiotics in agriculture and the risk to human health: How worried should we be? " *Evolutionary Applications*. August 2.

Chapman, H. D., & Z. B. Johnson. (2002). "Use of Antibiotics and Roxarsone in Broiler Chickens in the USA: Analysis for the Years 1995 to 2000," *Poultry Science*, *81*,356-64.

Choct, M. (2001). "Alternatives to in-feed antibiotics in monogastric animal industry," American Soybean Association Technical Bulletin. No. 217/10/2000 AN30-2001. pp. 1-6.

Clifford, Stephanie. (2008). "Tyson Told to End an Antibiotic Claim." *New York Times*, April 23. Cohen, M.L., and R.V. Tauxe. 1986. "Drug-Resistant Salmonella in the United States: An Epidemiologic Perspective," *Science*, *234*, 964-69.

Consumer Reports. (2012). Meat on Drugs: The Overuse of Antibiotics in Food Animals and What Supermarkets and Consumers Can Do to Stop It. Yonkers, NY. http://www.consumerreports.org/content/dam/cro/news_articles/health/CR%20Meat%20On%20Drugs%20Report%2006-12.pdf.

Consumers Union. Undated. The Overuse of Antibiotics in Food Animals Threatens Public Health. https://consumersunion.org/news/the-overuse-of-antibiotics-in-food-animals-threatens-public-health-2/.

Council for Agricultural Science and Technology (CAST). (1981). *Antibiotics in Animal Feeds*. Report No. 88. March. Ames, Iowa.

Cromwell, G. L. (1991). "Antimicrobial Agents." *Swine Nutrition*. Eds.: E.R. Miller, D.E. Ullrey, and A.J. Lewis, pp. 297-314. Boston: Butterworth-Heinemann.

Cromwell, G. L. (2002). "Why and how antibiotics are used in swine production," *Anima Biotechnology*, *13*(1), 7-27.

Danish Integrated Antimicrobial Resistance Monitoring and Research Program (DANMAP). (1999). Consumption of antimicrobial agents and occurrence of antimicrobial resistance in bacteria from food animals, food and humans in Denmark. Statens Serum Institut; Danish Medicines Agency; National Veterinary Institute, Technical University of Denmark; National Food Institute, Technical University of Denmark. http://www.danmap.org/~/media/Projekt%20sites/Danmap/DANMAP%20reports/Danmap_1999. ashx.

Danish Integrated Antimicrobial Resistance Monitoring and Research Program (DANMAP). 2010. Use of antimicrobial agents and occurrence of antimicrobial resistance in bacteria from food animals, food and humans in Denmark. Statens Serum Institut; Danish Medicines Agency; National Veterinary Institute, Technical University of Denmark; National Food Institute, Technical University of Denmark. http://www.danmap.org/~/media/Projekt%20sites/Danmap/DANMAP%20reports/Danmap_2010.ashx.

Danish Integrated Antimicrobial Resistance Monitoring and Research Program (DANMAP). 2011. Use of antimicrobial agents and occurrence of antimicrobial resistance in bacteria from food animals, food and humans in Denmark. Statens Serum Institut; Danish Medicines Agency; National Veterinary Institute, Technical University of Denmark; National Food Institute, Technical University of Denmark. http://www.danmap.org/~/media/Projekt%20sites/Danmap/DANMAP%20reports/Danmap_2011.ashx.

Danish Integrated Antimicrobial Resistance Monitoring and Research Program (DANMAP). 2012. Use of antimicrobial agents and occurrence of antimicrobial resistance in bacteria from food animals, food and humans in Denmark. Statens Serum Institut; Danish Medicines Agency; National Veterinary Institute, Technical University of Denmark; National Food Institute, Technical University of Denmark. http://www.danmap.org/~/media/Projekt%20sites/Danmap/DANMAP%20reports/DANMAP%202012/Danmap_2012.ashx.

Dibner, J. J. & J. D. Richards. (2005). "Antibiotic growth promoters in agriculture: History and mode of action," *Poultry Science*, *84*, 634-43.

Doyle, M. E. (2001). "Alternatives to antibiotic use for growth promotion in animal husbandry," Food Research Institute Briefing. April.

Dritz, S. S., Tokach, M. D., Goodband, R. D. & Nelssen, J. L. (2002). "Effects of administration of antimicrobials in feed on growth rate and feed efficiency of pigs in multisite production system," *Journal of the American Veterinary Medical Association*, *220*(11), 1690-95.

Dworkin, F. H. (1976). Some economic consequences of restricting the subtherapeutic use of tetracycline in feedlot cattle and swine. Office of Planning and Evaluation, Food and Drug Administration. OPE Study 33. November.

Engster, H. M., Marvil, D. & Stewart-Brown, B. (2002). "The effect of withdrawing growth promoting antibiotics from broiler chickens: A long-term commercial industry study," *Journal of Applied Poultry Research*, *11*, 431-36.

Emborg, H. D., Ersboll, A. K., Heuer, O.E. & Wegener, H.C. (2001). "The effect of discontinuing the use of antimicrobial growth promoters on the productivity in the Danish broiler productions," *Preventive Veterinary Medicine*, *50*(1), 53-70.

European Agency for the Evaluation of Medicinal Products. (1999). Antibiotic resistance in the European Union associated with therapeutic use of veterinary medicines. Report and qualitative risk assessment. Committee for Veterinary Medicinal Products. July 14.

Food and Agriculture Organization of the United Nations (FAO). (2014). FAOSTAT. Production. Livestock Primary. http://faostat.fao.org/site/569/default.aspx#ancor. Accessed July 2, 2014.

Freese, M. (2013). "Top 25 U.S. Pork Powerhouses 2013," *Successful Farming*.
http://www.agriculture.com/uploads/assets/promo/external/pdf/PP2013_03.pdf.

Gilliam, H. C., & J. R. Martin. (1975). "Economic importance of antibiotics in feeds to producers and consumers of pork, beef and veal," *Journal of Animal Science*, *40*(6), 1241-55.

Graham, J. P., Boland, J. J. & Silbergeld, E. (2007). "Growth promoting antibiotics in food animal production: An economic analysis," *Public Health Reports*, *122*, 79-87.

Greene, C. (2014). "Support for the Organic Sector Expands in the 2014 Farm Act. *Amber Waves*. ERS USDA. July. http://www.ers.usda.gov/amber-waves/2014-july/support-for-the-organic-sector-expands-in-the-2014-farm-act.aspx#.VfG1ypiFNGF.

Harrison, E. M., Paterson, G. K., Holden, M. T. G., Larsen, J., Stegger, M., Larsen, A. R., Petersen, A., Skov, R. L., Christensen, J. M., Zeuthen, A. V., Heltberg, O., Harris, S. R., Zadoks, R. N., Parkhill, J., Peacock, S. J. & Holmes. M. A. (2013). "Whole genome sequencing identifies zoonotic transmission of MRSA isolates with the novel MecA homologue mecC," *EMBO Molecular Medicine*, (Summer 2013), 509-15.

Hayes, D. J., Jensen, H. H., Backstrom, L. & Fabiosa, J. (1999). Economic Impact of a Ban on the Use of Over-the-Counter Antibiotics in U.S. Swine Rations. Center for Agricultural and Rural Development Staff Report 99 SR 90. December. Iowa State University, Ames, IA.

Hayes, D. J., Jensen, H. H., Backstrom, L. & Fabiosa. J. (2001). "Economic impact of a ban on the use of over-the-counter antibiotics in U.S. swine rations," *International Food and Agribusiness Management Review*, Special Issue: Private Sector Management of Food Safety, *4*(1), 81-97.

Hays, V. W. (1991). "Effects of antibiotics." In: Growth Regulation in Farm Animals. Advances in Meat Research. Vol. 7. A.M. Pearson and T.R. Dutson, eds. Pp. 299-320. New York: Elsevier Applied Science.

Headley, J. C. (1978). "Economic aspects of drug and chemical feed additives." Paper prepared for the Office of Technology Assessment, U.S. Congress. Washington, DC: U.S. Government Printing Office.

Hogberg, M. G., Raper, K. C. & Oehmke. J. F. (2009). "Banning subtherapeutic antibiotics in U.S. swine production: A simulation of impacts on industry structure." *Agribusiness*, *25*(3), 314-30.

Holmberg, S. D., Wells, J. G. & Cohen, M. L. (1984). "Animal-to-Man Transmission of Antimicrobial- Resistant Salmonella: Investigations of U.S. Outbreaks, 1971-1983," *Science*, *225*, 833-35. August.

Hughes, P. & Heritage, J. (2004). "Antibiotic Growth-Promoters in Food Animals." Food and Agriculture Organization of the United Nations.

Animal Production and Health Paper. http://www.fao.org/docrep/ARTICLE/AGRIPPA/555_EN.HTM.

Infectious Diseases Society of America. 2010. Statement on: Antibiotic Resistance: Promoting Judicious Use of Medically Important Antibiotics in Animal Agriculture before the House Committee on Energy and Commerce Subcommittee on Health. July 14. http://www.idsociety.org/uploadedFiles/IDSA/Policy_and_Advocacy/Current_ Topics_and_Issues/Advancing_Product_Research_and_Development/Vaccines/Statements/Testimony%20on%20Judicious%20Use%20of%20Antibiotics%20in%20Animals%20House%20EC%20Subcommittee%20on%20Health%20071410.pdf.

Institute of Medicine. (1988). Report of a Study: Human Health Risks with the Subtherapeutic Use of Penicillin or Tetracyclines in Animal Feed. Committee on Human Health. Washington, DC: National Academies Press.

Institute of Medicine. (2003). Microbial Threats to Health: Emergence, Detection, and Response. Committee on Emerging Microbial Threats to Health in the 21st Century. Washington, DC: National Academies Press.

Jensen, H. H. & Hayes, D. J. (2014). "Impact of Denmark's ban on antimicrobials for growth promotion," *Current Opinion in Microbiology*, *19*, 30-36.

Johnson, R. (2011). Potential Trade Implications of Restrictions on Antimicrobial Use in Animal Production. Congressional Research Service (CRS) Report for Congress July 11. 7-5700. R41047.

Joint Committee on the use of Antibiotics in Animal Husbandry and Veterinary Medicine. (1969). Report Presented to Parliament by the Secretary of State for Social Services, the Secretary of State for Scotland, the Minister of Agriculture, Fisheries and Food and the Secretary of State for Wales by Command of Her Majesty. November.

Key, N. & McBride, W. D. (2013). *U.S. Hog Production from 1992 to 2009: Technology, Restructuring, and Productivity Growth.* USDA, Economic Research Service, Economic Research Report (ERR-158). October.

Key, N. & McBride, W. D. (2014). "Sub-therapeutic antibiotics and the efficiency of U.S. hog farms," *American Journal of Agricultural Economics*, *96*(3), 831-50.

Khan, A. (2010). Statements to the House, Committee on Energy and Commerce, Subcommittee on Health re "Antibiotic Resistance and the Use of Antibiotics in Animal Agriculture." Hearing, July 14.

Kjeldsen, N. (2002). "Producing pork without antibiotic growth promoters: The Danish experience." *Advances in Pork Production*, *13*, 107-15. Online. Available at http://www.banffpork.ca/proc/2002pdf/BO04 Kjeldsen.pdf.

Larsen, P. B. (2002). "Consequences of termination of AGP use for pig health and usage of anti-microbials for therapy and prophylaxis." In: International Invitational Symposium; Beyond Antimicrobial Growth Promoters in Food Animal Production, November 6-7, 2002, Foulum, Denmark.

Lawrence, R. S. (2012). "The FDA did not do enough to restrict antibiotics use in animals," *The Atlantic.* Apr. 16. Available at http://www.theatlantic.com/health/archive/2012/04/ the-fda-did-not-do-enough-to-restrict-antibiotics-use-in-animals/255878/.

Lawrence, J. D. & Ibarburu, M. A. (2007). "Economic analysis of pharmaceutical technologies in modern beef production." Proceedings of the NCCC-134 Conference on Applied Commodity Price Analysis, Forecasting, and Market Risk Management. Chicago, IL.

Lawson, L. G., Jensen, F.V. & Otto, L. (2008). "The economics of use and non-use of antimicrobial growth promoters: The case of Danish broiler production," *Journal of International Farm Management*, *4*(2).

Levy, S. (2014). "Reduced antibiotic use in livestock: How Denmark tackled resistance." *Environmental Health Perspectives* News: Spheres of Influence 122(6). http:// ehp.niehs.nih. gov/122-a160/#r12.

Liu, X., Miller, G.Y. & McNamara, P. E. (2005). "Do antibiotics reduce production risk for U.S. pork producers? " *Journal of Agriculture and Applied Economics.*, *27*(December), 565-75.

Loglisci, R. (2010). "New FDA numbers reveal food animals consume lion's share of antibiotics." Johns Hopkins Bloomberg School of Public Health's Center for a Livable Future blog. http://www.livablefutureblog.com/ 2010/12/new-fda-numbers-reveal-food-animals-consume-lion%E2%80%99s-share-of-antibiotics.

Lusk, J. L., Norwood, F. B. & Pruitt, J. B. (2006). "Consumer demand for a ban on antibiotic drug use in pork production," *American Journal of Agricultural Economics*, *88*(4), 1015-33.

MacDonald, J. M. (2014). Technology, Organization, and Financial Performance in U.S. Broiler Production. USDA, Economic Research Service, EIB-126. June.

MacDonald, J. M. & Wang, S. L. (2011). "Foregoing Sub-Therapeutic Antibiotics: The Impact on Broiler Grow-out Operations," *Applied Economic Perspectives and Policy*, *33*(1), 79-98.

Mann, T. & Paulsen, A. (1976). "Economic impact of restricting feed additives in livestock and poultry production," *American Journal of Agricultural Economics*, *58*, 47-53.

Mather, A. E., Reid, S. W. J., Maskell, D. J., Parkhill, J., Fookes, M. C., Harris, S. R., Brown, K. J., Coia, J. E., Mulvey, M. R., Gilmour, M. W., Petrovska, L., de Pinna, E., Kuroda, M., Akiba, M., Izumiya, H., Connor, T. R., Suchard, M. A., Lemey, P., Mellor, D. J., Haydon, D. T. & Thomson, N. R. (2013). "Distinguishable Epidemics of Multidrug-Resistant Salmonella Typhimurium DT104 in Different Hosts," *Sciencexpress*, September 12, 1-8.

Mathews, K. H. (2001). *Antimicrobial Drug Use and Veterinary Costs in U.S. Livestock Production*. USDA, Economic Research Service, Agricultural Information Bulletin (AIB-766).

Mathew, K. H. (2002). "Economic effects of a ban against antimicrobial drugs used in U.S. beef production" *Journal of Agricultural and Applied Economics*, *34*(3), 513-30.

Maves, M. D. (2009). Letter to The Honorable Louise Slaughter, U.S. House of Representatives. American Medical Association. April 9. http://www.keepantibiotics-working.com/new/KAWfiles/64_2_106530.pdf.

McBride, W. D., Key, N. & Mathews, K. H. (2008). "Subtherapeutic antibiotics and productivity in U.S. hog production," *Review of Agricultural Economics*, *30*(2), 270-88.

McDonald's Corporation. (2003). "McDonald's Global Policy on Antibiotic Use in Food Animals." http://www.aboutmcdonalds.com/content/dam/AboutMcDonalds/Sustainability/Sustainability%20Library/antibiotics_policy.pdf.

——— 2015. "McDonald's USDA Announces New Antibiotics Policy and Menu Sourcing Initiatives." http://news.mcdonalds.com/Corporate/news-stories/McDonald-s-USA-Announces-New-Antibiotics-Policy-an.

McEwen, S. A. & Fedorka-Cray, P. J. (2002). "Antimicrobial Use and Resistance in Animals," *Clinical Infectious Diseases*, *34*(Suppl. 3), S93-106.

Mellon, M. (2013). "Negotiating with drug companies: The horse-trading behind the FDA's voluntary program." The Equation. Union of Concerned

Scientists. http://blog.ucsusa. org/negotiating-with-drug-companies-the-horse-trading-behind-the-fdas-voluntary-program.

Miller, G. Y., Liu, X., McNamara, P. E. & Bush, E. J. (2005). "Farm-level impacts of banning growth promoting antibiotic use in U.S. Pig Grower/Finisher Operations," *Journal of Agribusiness*, *23*(Fall), 147-62.

Morley, P. S., Margate, D. A., Hyatt, D. R., Dewell, G. A., Patterson, J. G., Burgess, B. A. & Wittum, T. E. (2011) "Effects of restricted antimicrobial exposure on antimicrobial resistance in fecal Escherichia Coli from feedlot cattle," *Foodborne Pathogens and Disease*, *8*(1), 87-98.

Muth, M. K., Beach, R. H. Shawn, A. K., Taylor, J. L. & Viator, C. L. (2006). "Poultry Slaughter and Processing Sector Facility-Level Model." Final Report. Contract No. 53-3A94-03-12, Deliver Order 10, Prepared for Ronald L. Meekhof, USDA/FSIS/IPPED. Washington, DC. http://www.rti.org/pubs/poultry_slaughter.pdf.

Muth, M. K, Zhen, C., Beach, R. H., Karns, S. A., Taylor, J. L. & Viator, C. L. (2007). "Pork Slaughter and Processing Sector Facility-Level Model." Final Report. Contract No. 53-3A94-03-12, Delivery Order 9, Prepared for Ronald L. Meekhof, USDA/FSIS/OPPED. Washington, DC. http://www.rti.org/pubs/muth_pork-slaughter_final.pdf.

National Academy of Sciences. (1980). "The Effects on Human Health of Subtherapeutic Use of Antimicrobial Drugs in Animal Feeds." Committee to Study the Human Health Effects of Subtherapeutic Antibiotic Use in Animal Feeds. Washington, DC *National Hog Farmer*, 2011. "10 Crucial Steps to Sow and Litter Care." October 19th issue. http://nationalhogfarmer.com/health-diseases/10-crucial-steps-sow-care-1015.

National Research Council (NRC). (1999). *The Use of Drugs in Food Animals: Benefits and Risks*. Washington, DC: National Academies Press.

Nemechek, J. E., Tokach, M. D., Dritz, S. S., Goodband, R. D., DeRouchey, J. M. & Bergstrom, J. R. (2013). "Evaluation of antibiotics and benzoic acid on growth performance of nursery pigs," Paper presented at Swine Day Conference, Nov. 21. Manhattan, KS. http://krex.k-state.edu/dspace/handle/2097/17344.

Oliver, W. T. & Wells, J. E. (2013). "Lysozyme as an alternative to antibiotics improves growth promotion and small intestinal morphology in nursery pigs," *Journal of Animal Science*, *91*(7), 3129-36.

Osteen, C, J Gottlieb, Vasavada, U., Aillery, M., Beckman, A., Borchers, A., Classing, R., Day-Rubenstein, K., Ebel, R., Fernandez-Cornejo, J., Greene, C., Heisey, P., Hellerstein, D., Hoppe, R. Huang, W., Kuethe, T.,

Livingston, M., Nickerson, C., Ribaudo, M., Schaible, G. & Wang, S. L. (2012). *Agricultural Resources and Environmental Indicators 2012*, USDA, Economic Research Service, Economic Information Bulletin (EIB-98). August.

Pew Charitable Trusts. (2015). Top food companies moving away from overuse of antibiotics on industrial farms. March 9. http://www.pewtrusts.org/en/research-and-analysis/fact-sheets/2014 /04/09/top-food-companies-moving-away-from-overuse-of-antibiotics-on-industrial-farms.

Phillips, I., Casewell, M., Cox, T., De Groot, B., Friis, C., Jones, R., Nightingale, C., Preston, R. & Waddell, J. (2004). "Does the use of antibiotics in food animals pose a risk to human health? A critical review of published data," *Journal of Antimicrobial Chemotherapy*, *53*, 28-52.

Price, L. B., Stegger, M., Hasman, H., Aziz, M., Larsen, J., Andersen, P. S., Pearson, T., Waters, A. E., Foster, J. T., Schupp, J., Gillece, J., Driebe, Liu, C. M., Springer, B. Zdovc, I., Battisti, A., Franco, A., Zmudski, J., Schwarz, S., Butaye, P., Jouy, E., Pomba, C., Porrero, M. C., Remy, R., Smith, T. C., Robinson, D. A., Weese, J. S., Arriola, C. S., Yu, F., Laurent, F., Keim, P., Skov, R. & Aarestrup, F. M., (2012). "Staphylococcus aureus CC398: Host Adaptation and Emergence of Methicillin Resistance in Livestock," *mBio*, *3*(1), 1-6.

Raymond, R. (2013). "Antibiotics and animals raised for food: Lies, damn lies and statistics." Food Safety News. January 7. http://www.foodsafety news.com/2013/01/antibiotics-and-animals-raised-for-food-lies-damn-lies-and-statistics/#.VK2uXSvF98E.

Robertsson, J. A. & Lundeheim, N. (1994). Prohibited use of antibiotics as a feed additive for growth promotion – effects on piglet health and production parameters. In Proceedings of the International Pig Vet. Soc. Congress (p. 282). Bangkok, Thailand.

Seattle-King County Department of Public Health. (1984). "Surveillance of the Flow of Salmonella and Campylobacter in a Community." Prepared for United States Department of Health and Human Services, Public Health Service, Food and Drug Administration, Bureau of Veterinary Medicine. Contract Number 223-81-7041.

Sharfstein, Joshua. (2010). Statements to the House, Committee on Energy and Commerce, Subcommittee on Health, re "Antibiotic Resistance and the Use of Antibiotics in Animal Agriculture." Hearing, July 14.

Shea, K. M. (2004). "Nontherapeutic use of antimicrobial agents in animal agriculture: Implication for pediatrics." American Academy of Pediatrics Technical Report. *Pediatrics, 114*(3), 862-68.

Smith, J. A. (2011). "Experiences with drug-free broiler production," *Poultry Science* 90:2670-78. Turnidge, J. 2004a. "Antibiotic use in animals – prejudices, perceptions and realities," *Journal of Antimicrobial Chemotherapy, 53*, 26-27.

Turnidge, J. (2004b). "Reply," in *Journal of Antimicrobial Chemotherapy* 53(5):886.

U.S. Centers for Disease Control and Prevention (CDC). (2013). Antibiotic Resistance Threats in the United States, 2013. http://www.cdc.gov/drugresistance/threat-report-2013/pdf/ar-threats-2013-508.pdf.

U.S. Department of Agriculture. (1978). *Economic effects of a prohibition on the use of selected animal drugs.* Economics, Statistics, and Cooperatives Service. Agricultural Economic Report (AER-414). Washington, DC. November.

U.S. Department of Agriculture (USDA), Animal and Plant Health Inspection Service (APHIS). (2002). *Swine 2000, Part II: Reference of Swine Health and Management in the United States,2000.* USDA-APHIS-VS, CEAH, Fort Collins, CO. #N355.0202.

U.S. Department of Agriculture (USDA), Animal and Plant Health Inspection Service (APHIS). (2007a). *Dairy 2007, Part I: Reference of Dairy Cattle Health and Management Practices in the United States, 2007.* USDA-APHIS-VS, CEAH. Fort Collins, CO. #N480.1007.

U.S. Department of Agriculture (USDA), Animal and Plant Health Inspection Service (APHIS). (2007b). *Swine 2006, Part II: Reference of Swine Health and Health Management Practices in theUnited States, 2006.* USDA:APHIS:VS, CEAH. Fort Collins, CO. #N479.1007.

U.S. Department of Agriculture (USDA), Animal and Plant Health Inspection Service (APHIS). (2007c). *Swine 2006, Part III: Reference of Swine Health and Management Practices in theUnited States, 2006.* USDA:APHIS:VS, CEAH. Fort Collins, CO. #N475.1007.

U.S. Department of Agriculture (USDA), Animal and Plant Health Inspection Service (APHIS). (2008). *Dairy 2007, Part III: Reference of Dairy Cattle Health and Management Practices in the United States, 2007.* USDA-APHIS-VS, CEAH. Fort Collins, CO. #N482.0908.

U.S. Department of Agriculture (USDA), Animal and Plant Health Inspection Service (APHIS). (2010). *Beef 2007-08 Part IV: Reference of Beef Cow-*

calf Management Practices in the United States, 2007-08. Fort Collins, CO, #523.0210.

U.S. Department of Agriculture, Animal and Plant Health Inspection Service (APHIS). (2012). *Dairy Heifer Raiser, 2011. An overview of operations that specialize in raising dairy heifers.* USDA- APHIS-VS, CEAH, National Animal Health Monitoring System (NAHMS), Fort Collins, CO.#613.1012.

U.S. Department of Agriculture (USDA), Animal and Plant Health Inspection Service (APHIS). (2013)a. Feedlot 2011 *"Part I: Management Practices on U.S. Feedlots with a Capacity of 1,000 or More Head."* USDA-APHIS-VS-CEAH-NAHMS. Fort Collins, CO. #626.0313.

U.S. Department of Agriculture (USDA), Animal and Plant Health Inspection Service (APHIS). (2013b). Feedlot 2011 *"Part II: Management Practices on U.S. Feedlots with a Capacity of Fewer than 1,000 Head."* USDA-APHIS-VS-CEAH-NAHMS. Fort Collins, CO. #626.0313.

U.S. Department of Agriculture (USDA), Animal and Plant Health Inspection Service (APHIS). (2013c). Feedlot 2011 *"Part III: Trends in Health and Management Practices on U.S. Feedlots, 1994-2011."* USDA-APHIS-VS-CEAH-NAHMS. Fort Collins, CO.

U.S. Department of Agriculture (USDA), Economic Research Service (ERS). (2014a). Food Availability (Per Capita) Data System. Food Availability: Red meat (beef, veal, pork, lamb, and mutton). http://www.ers.usda.gov/data-products/food-availability-(per-capita)-data-system/.aspx#.U4zgVPldXep.

U.S. Department of Agriculture (USDA), Economic Research Service (ERS). (2014b). Pork values and spreads. http://www.ers.usda.gov/data-products/meat-price-spreads. aspx#.U4zeovldXeq.

U.S. Department of Agriculture (USDA), Economic Research Service (ERS). (2014c). Food Availability (Per Capita) Data System. Food Availability: Poultry (chicken and turkey). http://www.ers.usda.gov/data-products/food-availability-(per-capita)-data-system/.aspx#. U4zgVPldXep.

U.S. Department of Agriculture (USDA), Economic Research Service (ERS). (2014d). Retail prices for beef, pork, poultry cuts, eggs, and dairy products. http://www.ers.usda.gov/data-products/meat-price-spreads.aspx #.U4zhG_ldXer.

U.S. Department of Agriculture (USDA), Food Safety and Inspection Service (FSIS). (2013). United States National Residue Program for Meat, Poultry, and Egg Products. 2011 Residue Sample Results. Office of Public

Health Science. http://www.fsis.usda.gov/wps/ wcm/connect/f511ad0e-d148-4bec-95c7-22774e731f7c/2011_Red_Book.pdf?MOD =AJPERES.

U.S. Department of Agriculture (USDA), Grain Inspection, Packers and Stockyards Administration (GIPSA). (2014). 2013 Annual Report, Packers and Stockyards Program. March. http://www.gipsa.usda.gov/Publications/psp/ar/2013_psp_annual_report.pdf.

U.S. Department of Agriculture (USDA), National Agricultural Statistics Service (NASS). (2004). Quarterly Hogs and Pigs. December 28. Washington, DC. http://usda.mannlib.cornell.edu/usda/nass/HogsPigs//2000s/2004/HogsPigs-12-28-2004.pdf.

U.S. Department of Agriculture (USDA), National Agricultural Statistics Service (NASS). (2009). Quarterly Hogs and Pigs. December 30. Washington, DC. http://usda.mannlib.cornell.edu/usda/nass/HogsPigs//2000s/2009/HogsPigs-12-30-2009.pdf.

U.S. Department of Agriculture (USDA), National Agricultural Statistics Service (NASS). (2005). Farms, Land in Farms, and Livestock Operations, 2004 Summary. January. Sp Sy 5 (05). http://usda.mannlib.cornell.edu/usda/nass/FarmLandIn//2000s/2005/FarmLandIn-01-31-2005.pdf.

U.S. Department of Agriculture (USDA), National Agricultural Statistics Service (NASS). (2010). Farms, Land in Farms, and Livestock Operations, 2009 Summary. February. Sp Sy 5 (10) a. http://usda.mannlib.cornell.edu/usda/nass/FarmLandIn//2010s/2010/FarmLandIn-02-12-2010_revision.pdf.

U.S. Department of Agriculture (USDA), National Agricultural Statistics Service (NASS). (2013a). Farms, Land in Farms, and Livestock Operations, 2012 Summary. February. http://usda.mannlib.cornell.edu/usda/nass/FarmLandIn//2010s/2013/FarmLandIn-02-19-2013.pdf.

U.S. Department of Agriculture (USDA), National Agricultural Statistics Service (NASS). (2013b). Milk Production. Dec. 19. http://usda.mannlib.cornell.edu/usda/nass/MilkProd//2010s/2013/MilkProd-12-19-2013.pdf.

U.S. Department of Agriculture (USDA), National Agricultural Statistics Service (NASS). (2014a). Quarterly Hogs and Pigs. March 28. http://usda.mannlib.cornell.edu/usda/nass/HogsPigs//2010s/2014/HogsPigs-03-28-2014.pdf.

U.S. Department of Agriculture (USDA), National Agricultural Statistics Service (NASS). (2014b). 2012 Agricultural Census. United States Summary and State Data. Volume 1, Geographic Area Series. Part 51. http://www.agcensus.usda.gov/Publications/2012/ Full_Report/Volume_1,_Chapter_1_US/usv1.pdf.

U.S. Department of Agriculture, National Agricultural Statistics Service (NASS). (2014c). Cattle on Feed, February 21, http://usda.mannlib .cornell.edu/usda/nass/CattOnFe// 2010s/2014/CattOnFe-02-21-2014.pdf.

U.S. Department of Agriculture (USDA), National Agricultural Statistics Service (NASS). (2015). Milk Production. Released Feb. 20. http://usda.mannlib.cornell.edu/usda/current/ MilkProd/MilkProd-02-20-2015.pdf.

U.S. Food and Drug Administration (FDA). (2003). *Guidance for Industry: Evaluating the Safety of Antimicrobial New Animal Drugs with Regard to Their Microbiological Effects on Bacteria of Human Health Concern.* Department of Health and Human Services, Center for Veterinary Medicine. #152.

U.S. Food and Drug Administration (FDA). (2011). Grade "A" Pasteurized Milk Ordinance. 2011 Revision. Department of Health and Human Services. Public Health Service. http://www.fda.gov/downloads/Food/ GuidanceRegulation/UCM291757.pdf.

U.S. Food and Drug Administration (FDA). (2012a). *Guidance for Industry: The Judicious Use of Medically Important Antimicrobial Drugs in Food-Producing Animals.* Department of Health and Human Services Center for Veterinary Medicine. #209.

U.S. Food and Drug Administration (FDA). (2012b). *National Antimicrobial Resistance Monitoring System – Enteric Bacteria (NARMS). 2010 Executive Report.* Rockville, MD: U.S. Department of Health and Human Services, Food and Drug Administration.

U.S. Food and Drug Administration (FDA). (2012c). Estimates of antibacterial drug sales in human medicine. http://www.fda.gov/Drugs/DrugSafety InformationbyDrugClass/ ucm261160.htm.

U.S. Food and Drug Administration (FDA). (2013). *Guidance for Industry: New Animal Drugs and New Animal Drug Combination Products Administered in or on Medicated Feed or Drinking Water of Food-Producing Animals: Recommendations for Drug Sponsors for Voluntarily Aligning Product Use Conditions with GFI # 209.* #213.

U.S. Food and Drug Administration (FDA). (2014a). "From an Idea to the Marketplace: The Journey of an Animal Drug through the Approval

Process." June. Department of Health and Human Services. http://www.fda.gov/AnimalVeterinary/ResourcesforYou/Animal HealthLiteracy/ucm219207.htm.

U.S. Food and Drug Administration (FDA). 2014b. National Antimicrobial Resistance Monitoring System. Introduction to NARMS. July. http://www.fda.gov/animal veterinary/safetyhealth/antimicrobialresistance /nationalantimicrobialresistance monitoringsystem/default.htm.

U.S. Food and Drug Administration (FDA). (2014c). "FDA secures full industry engagement on anti-microbial resistance strategy." June 30. Department of Health and Human Services. http://www.fda.gov/ AnimalVeterinary/NewsEvents/CVMUpdates/ucm 403285. htm.

U.S. Government Accountability Office (GAO). (1999). *Food Safety: The Agricultural Use of Antibiotics and Its Implications for Human Health.* Report to the Honorable Tom Harkin, Ranking Minority Member, Committee on Agriculture, Nutrition, and Forestry, U.S. Senate. April. GAO/RCED-88-74.

U.S. Government Accountability Office (GAO). (2011). *Antibiotic resistance: Agencies have made limited progress addressing antibiotic use in animals.* GAO-11-801. Report to the Ranking Member, Committee on Rules, House of Representatives.

Wade, M. A., & Barkley, A. P. (1992). "The economic impacts of a ban on subtherapeutic antibiotics in swine production," *Agribusiness*, *8*, 93-107.

Weise, E. (2006). " 'Natural' chickens take flight," *USA Today*, Jan. 23. D5.

Wierup, M. (2001). "The Swedish experience of the 1986 year ban of antimicrobial growth promoters, with special reference to animal health, disease prevention, productivity, and usage of antimicrobials," *Microbiotic Drug Resistance*, *7*(2), 183-190.

World Health Organization (WHO). (1997). The Medical Impact of Antimicrobial Use in Food Animals. Report of a WHO Meeting. Berlin, Germany, 13-17 October. http://whqlibdoc.who.int/hq/1997/WHO_EMC_ ZOO_97.4.pdf.

World Health Organization (WHO). (2000). WHO Global Principles for the Containment of Antimicrobial Resistance in Animals Intended for Food. Report of a WHO Consultation with the participation of the Food and Agriculture Organization of the United Nations and the Office International des Epizooties. Geneva, Switzerland. June 5-9. http://whqlibdoc.who.int/hq/2000/WHO_CDS_CSR_APH_2000.4.pdf.

World Health Organization (WHO). (2002). *Impacts of antimicrobial growth promoter termination in Denmark.* The WHO international review panel's

evaluation of the termination of the use of anti-microbial growth promoters in Denmark. Foulum, Denmark. November. 6-9.
World Health Organization (WHO). 2012. *The Evolving Threat of Antimicrobial Resistance: Options for Action.* Geneva, Switzerland. http://whqlibdoc.who.int/publications/ 2012/9789241503181_eng.pdf.

End Notes

[1] "Medically important" antibiotics are those important for treating human disease. A list of medically important antibiotics can be found in U.S.FDA, 2003.

[2] Amounts that consumers *say* in a survey that they would be willing to pay for a specific food attribute may differ from what they will *actually* pay when making purchasing decisions.

[3] Caveats to this practice were that this only applied to antibiotics used in human medicine and referred only to situations in which McDonald's "has a direct relationship in the meat purchasing supply chain process."

[4] While scours causes the most disease-induced death in preweaned piglets, crushing by sow and piglets refusing to eat cause a higher percentage of deaths (42.0 and 29.7 percent, respectively).

[5] Recall that the NAHMS surveys operations with more than 100 head.

[6] Calculation of the percentage of hogs removed or sold that received antibiotics assumes that all nursery hogs at the operations administering antibiotics to nursery hogs received antibiotics for the stated purpose. This is in contrast to only a portion of hogs at an operation receiving antibiotics for the stated purpose. The latter is a safe assumption for administration of growth promotion and disease prevention, but is a strong assumption when referring to disease treatment. Thus, the percentage of hogs receiving antibiotics for disease treatment is likely less than 59 percent.

[7] As previously noted, the NAHMS includes operations with 100 or more head, while the ARMS samples operations with 25 or more head. The average operation size in the ARMS is therefore lower than that in the NAHMS, which may influence overall percentages. Restricting the ARMS sample to operations with at least 100 hogs slightly increases the percentage of operations reporting that they use antibiotics for growth promotion, from 33 to 34 percent. The "don't know" category rises from 8 to 9 percent.

[8] As noted in a prior section, data collection changes somewhat between 2004 and 2009. In 2004, respondents had the option to answer "yes" or "no" to questions on administration of antibiotics via feed or water; nonresponse was coded as "missing." In 2009, respondents were given the additional option of answering "don't know."

[9] One hypothesis for part of the jump in "don't know" respondents is the rise in contract production. Reporting of "don't know" is higher for contract operations; between 2004 and 2009 the percentage of contact production also grew. However, limiting respondents in both 2004 and 2009 to just contract producers yields qualitatively similar results, with similar increases in respondents in the "don't know/missing" category.

[10] Restricting the ARMS sample to operations with at least a 100-head inventory (to make the sample more comparable to NAHMS data) slightly increases the estimate of operations using antibiotics as growth promotants, from 30 to 34 percent, with the "don't know" category rising from 16 to 18 percent.

[11] "Cattle" is a generic term that can refer to all categories of bulls, steers, cows, heifers, and/or calves. A bull is a sexually mature, uncastrated male, generally employed for breeding purposes. A steer is a bovine male castrated before reaching sexual maturity. A cow is a mature female, usually having had at least one calf. A heifer is a bovine female that has not

given birth to a calf. Feeder cattle are usually yearling (between 1 and 2 years old) steers and/or heifers ready to be finished for market. Finishing is the stage of production prior to slaughter in which an animal's weight is increased to produce desirable carcass characteristics. These and other definitions can be found at: http://www.ers.usda.gov/topics/animal-products/animal-production-marketing-issues/glossary.aspx.

[12] As noted previously, ionophores and coccidiostats are two types of antimicrobials not used in human medicine.

[13] In an earlier survey of feedlots with 1,000 head or more, APHIS (2000) reported that only 2 antibiotics were fed for most of the feeding period (i.e., more than 30 days): Tylosin (fed for a feedlot average range of 138 to 145 days) and Virginiamycin (fed for 124.5 to 130 days). Of the two, only Tylosin is "related" to antibiotics used in human health care.

[14] There were about 9.22 million milk cows in 2013. To maintain this herd size nationwide, nearly 30 percent (2.77 million) of milk cows must be replaced in a year due to onsite deaths as well as to the culling of cows with reduced production. If replacement heifers enter the milking herd at around 24 months, the U.S. dairy sector will need to have 5.54 million replacement heifers on hand. Since some heifers die before entering the milking herd, the national herd of replacement heifers must be about 6 million animals. The estimate of the national milking herd is from USDA, NASS (2013b). Estimates of culling and mortality rates are drawn from the 2010 ARMS (Agricultural Resource Management Survey), version3.

[15] Note that heifers can be fed more than one medication; hence, percentages add to more than 100.

[16] These studies find that growth-promoting antibiotic use increased individual farm profits by $0.75 per pig marketed (2013$), or by 9 percent of returns for a typical grow-finish operation (Miller et al., 2005). Similar studies also find that antimicrobials fed for growth promotion decrease variability among hogs and therefore increase profits by $1,670 per operation (2013$). Note that in calculating these estimates, these studies assume no wide-scale changes in production- purpose antibiotic use (as would occur with a ban).

[17] In Monte Carlo simulation, the researcher specifies distributions of unknown parameters. In a single simulation, values from these distributions are randomly selected (by computer) and then used to calculate the outcomes. We specify parameter distributions for the elasticities of supply and demand, the percentage of production receiving production-purpose antibiotics, and the supply effects from restrictions on production-purpose antibiotic use (Table 22). In a single simulation of the pork market, a value between 1 and 3 is chosen as the supply effect, a value between 36 and 59 percent is chosen as the proportion of producers using production-purpose antibiotics, a value between 0.487 and 0.813 as the elasticity of supply, and a value between -0.794 and -0.467 as the elasticity of demand. The simulation is conducted many times, with each simulation using different values of the four parameters within specified ranges. The results of the multiple simulations can be summarized with average values and standard deviations of the outcomes. We repeat the Monte Carlo simulation 10,000 times and report the means and standard deviations of the estimated outcomes from the multiple simulations.

In: Antibiotic Use in U.S. Livestock Production ISBN: 978-1-63485-056-8
Editor: Karin Greer

Chapter 2

GUIDANCE FOR INDUSTRY: THE JUDICIOUS USE OF MEDICALLY IMPORTANT ANTIMICROBIAL DRUGS IN FOOD-PRODUCING ANIMALS*

Food and Drug Administration

This guidance represents the Food and Drug Administration's (FDA) current thinking on this topic. It does not create or confer any rights for or on any person and does not operate to bind FDA or the public. You can use an alternative approach if the approach satisfies the requirements of the applicable statutes and regulations. If you want to discuss an alternative approach, contact the FDA staff responsible for implementing this guidance. If you cannot identify the appropriate FDA staff, call the number listed on the previous page of this guidance.

I. EXECUTIVE SUMMARY

Antimicrobial drugs have been widely used in human and veterinary medicine for more than 50 years, with tremendous benefits to both human and animal health. The development of resistance to this important class of drugs,

* This is an edited, reformatted and augmented version of guidance document #209, issued by the U.S. Food and Drug Administration, Center for Veterinary Medicine, April 13, 2012.

and the resulting loss of their effectiveness as antimicrobial therapies, poses a serious public health threat. Misuse and overuse of antimicrobial drugs creates selective evolutionary pressure that enables antimicrobial resistant bacteria to increase in numbers more rapidly than antimicrobial susceptible bacteria and thus increases the opportunity for individuals to become infected by resistant bacteria. Because antimicrobial drug use contributes to the emergence of drug resistant organisms, these important drugs must be used judiciously in both animal and human medicine to slow the development of resistance. Efforts have been made to promote the judicious use of these drugs in humans (see http://www.cdc.gov/getsmart/index.html) as well as in animals (see http://www.avma.org/issues/default.asp). Using these drugs judiciously means that unnecessary or inappropriate use should be avoided. The focus of this document is on the use of medically important antimicrobial drugs[1] in food-producing animals. Based on a consideration of the available scientific information, FDA is providing a framework for the voluntary adoption of practices to ensure the appropriate or judicious use of medically important antimicrobial drugs in food-producing animals. This framework includes the principles of phasing in such measures as 1) limiting medically important antimicrobial drugs to uses in food-producing animals that are considered necessary for assuring animal health; and 2) limiting such drugs to uses in food-producing animals that include veterinary oversight or consultation. Developing strategies for reducing antimicrobial resistance is critically important for protecting both public and animal health. Collaboration involving the public, the public health, animal health, and animal agriculture communities on the development and implementation of such strategies is needed to assure that the public health is protected while also assuring that such strategies are feasible and that the health needs of animals are addressed.

FDA's guidance documents, including this guidance, do not establish legally enforceable responsibilities. Instead, guidances describe the Agency's current thinking on a topic and should be viewed only as recommendations, unless specific regulatory or statutory requirements are cited. The use of the word "should" in Agency guidances means that something is suggested or recommended, but not required.

II. Introduction

Antimicrobial resistance[2], and the resulting failure of antimicrobial therapies in humans, is a mounting public health problem of global significance. This phenomenon is driven by many factors including the use of antimicrobial drugs in both humans and animals. In regard to animal use, this document addresses the use of medically important antimicrobial drugs in food-producing animals for production or growth-enhancing purposes. These uses, referred to as production[3] uses throughout this document, are typically administered through the feed or water on a herd- or flock-wide basis and are approved for such uses as increasing rate of weight gain or improving feed efficiency. Unlike other uses of these drugs in animals (e.g., for the treatment, control, and prevention of disease), these "production uses" are not intended to manage a specific disease that may be ongoing or at risk of occurring, but rather are expressly indicated and used for the purpose of enhancing the production of animal-derived products (e.g., increasing rate of weight gain or improving feed efficiency). This document summarizes some of the key reports and scientific literature related to the use of antimicrobial drugs in animal agriculture and outlines FDA's current thinking on strategies for assuring that medically important antimicrobial drugs are used judiciously in food-producing animals in order to help minimize antimicrobial resistance development. In finalizing this guidance, FDA has considered comments that were submitted to the docket, and other relevant information. If you have additional relevant information, please submit it to the docket at any time. We are particularly interested in any new information regarding the use of medically important antimicrobials in food-producing animals and its impact on the development of drug-resistant bacteria.

III. Key Reports and Peer-Reviewed Scientific Literature on the Issue

Questions regarding the use of antimicrobial drugs in food-producing animals have been raised and debated for many years. A variety of recognized international, governmental, and professional organizations have studied the issue. We have briefly summarized below the findings and recommendations from some of the notable reports that have addressed this issue over the past 40 years. These reports provide context to FDA's current thinking on this issue, and highlight the longstanding concerns that have been the subject of discussion in the scientific community as a whole.

We have also provided a list below of some of the more recent primary scientific literature that FDA has considered. This is not intended to represent an exhaustive summary of the scientific literature, but rather to highlight some of the more recent scientific research related to the use of antimicrobial drugs in animal agriculture and the impact of such use on antimicrobial resistance. We acknowledge that a significant body of scientific information exists, including some information that may present equivocal findings or contrary views.

Unless otherwise indicated, the page numbers cited in this section refer to the relevant page numbers in the referenced report. A complete list of the reports summarized in this section is provided at Section IX of this document.

Reports Prepared by Various International, Governmental, and Professional Organizations

1969 Report of the Joint Committee on the Use of Antibiotics in Animal Husbandry and Veterinary Medicine

In July 1968, a Joint Committee was established in the United Kingdom to obtain information regarding the use of antibiotics in animal husbandry and veterinary medicine, particularly with respect to antibiotic resistance. This report, often referred to as the "Swann Report," was presented to Parliament in November 1969 by the Secretary of State for Social Services, the Secretary of State for Scotland, the Minister of Agriculture, Fisheries and Food, and the Secretary of State for Wales. The report concluded that the administration of antimicrobials to food-producing animals, particularly at subtherapeutic levels, poses a hazard to human and animal health.

The report stated, "It is clear that there has been a dramatic increase over the years in the numbers of strains of enteric bacteria of animal origin which show resistance to one or more antibiotics. Further, these resistant strains are able to transmit this resistance to other bacteria. This resistance has resulted from the use of antibiotics for growth promotion and other purposes in farm livestock" [1]. The report also noted, "There is ample and incontrovertible evidence to show that man may commonly ingest enteric bacteria of animal origin" [1].

The report provided a number of recommendations including that only antimicrobials which "have little or no application as therapeutic agents in man or animals and will not impair the efficacy of a prescribed therapeutic drug or drugs through the development of resistant strains of organisms" should be used without prescription in animal feed [1]. Furthermore, the report concluded that antimicrobials used for therapeutic purposes in food-producing animals should remain available but only under veterinary supervision.

1970 FDA Task Force Report, "The Use of Antibiotics in Animal Feed"

In April 1970, FDA established a task force of scientists to undertake a comprehensive review of the use of antibiotics in animal feed [2]. The task force included ten specialists on infectious diseases and animal science from FDA, the National Institutes of Health, the U.S. Department of Agriculture, and the Centers for Disease Control and Prevention, as well as five consultants from universities and industry.

This task force acknowledged that the understanding at the time it conducted its study was that the use of antimicrobials in food-producing animals, especially in subtherapeutic amounts, was associated with the development of resistant bacteria, and that treated animals might serve as a reservoir of antimicrobial-resistant pathogens that could produce human disease.

The recommendations of the Task Force included that antimicrobial drugs used in human clinical medicine that failed to meet certain guidelines established by the Task Force should be prohibited from growth promotion and any subtherapeutic use in food-producing animals by certain dates. Furthermore, those antimicrobials that failed to meet the guidelines should be limited to short-term therapeutic use and use only by a veterinarian or on a veterinarian's prescription.

As a consequence of the 1970 Task Force report, requirements for data to address microbiological safety concerns for subtherapeutic uses of antimicrobials in food-producing animals were outlined in the Code of Federal Regulations (21 CFR 558.15). Sponsors of antibiotic products administered in animal feed for subtherapeutic purposes were required to submit study results demonstrating that their product did not promote bacterial drug resistance. Depending on the class of drug, sponsors were required to submit all information to the agency on the impact of their drug on enteric salmonella in treated animals by specific dates.

1980 National Academy of Sciences Report, "The Effects on Human Health of Subtherapeutic Use of Antimicrobial Drugs in Animal Feeds"

In 1977, FDA proposed to withdraw the new animal drug approvals for subtherapeutic uses of penicillin and tetracyclines in animal feed on the ground that evidence showed that these drugs, when used for such purposes in animal feed, had not been shown to be safe. These two drugs were chosen because of their importance in human medicine. The proposal was criticized because, at that time, there was not adequate epidemiological evidence (or only just-emerging evidence) to show that drug-resistant bacteria of animal origin were commonly transmitted to humans and caused serious illness. Subsequently, Congress directed FDA to conduct further studies related to the use of antimicrobials in animal feed and to hold in abeyance the implementation of the proposed antimicrobial withdrawal actions pending the outcome of these studies.

In accordance with Congress' directive to conduct further studies, FDA contracted with the National Academy of Science to conduct a study of the safety issues related to the use of antimicrobials in animal feed. In particular, FDA asked the National Academy of Science to: 1) study the human health effects of the subtherapeutic use of penicillin and tetracycline in animal feed; 2) review and analyze published and unpublished data relevant to assessing human health consequences of such use; 3) assess the scientific feasibility of additional epidemiological studies; and (4) make recommendations about additional research needed.

The National Academy of Sciences issued a study report in 1980. The study report concluded that a very limited amount of epidemiological research had been completed on either the subtherapeutic or therapeutic use of antimicrobials in animal feed. According to the study report, much of the information available on the subject involved "poorly controlled studies of small numbers of subjects for brief periods" [3]. Based on a consideration of available evidence, the report concluded that existing data could neither prove nor disprove the postulated hazards to human health from subtherapeutic antimicrobial use in animal feed. However, the report cautioned that "The lack of data linking human illness with subtherapeutic levels of antimicrobials must not be equated with proof that the proposed hazards do not exist. The research necessary to establish and measure a definitive risk has not been conducted and, indeed, may not be possible" [3].

1984 Seattle-King County Study: "Surveillance of the Flow of Salmonella and Campylobacter in a Community"

As noted above, Congress directed FDA to hold in abeyance any implementation of the proposed withdrawal of new animal drug approvals for the subtherapeutic uses of penicillin and tetracyclines in animal feed, pending completion of additional studies related to the use of antimicrobials in animal feed. Therefore, in addition to the National Academy of Sciences study described above, the FDA also contracted with the Seattle-King County Health

Department to complete a study intended to provide additional information regarding potential public health concerns regarding the use of antimicrobial drugs in animal feed. Under the contract, the Communicable Disease Control Section of the Seattle-King County Health Department was tasked with studying the relationship between the occurrence of Salmonella spp. (*Salmonella*) and Campylobacter jejuni (*C. jejuni*) in foods of animal origin and the occurrence of human illness caused by those two organisms. These two organisms, *Salmonella* and *C. jejuni*, were chosen to serve as models to estimate the flow of potentially pathogenic bacteria from animals to man through the food chain. The study involved a two-pronged surveillance system that included sampling of retail meats over a 20 month period and simultaneous investigation of *Salmonella* and *C. jejuni* enteritis cases in humans. Bacterial isolates from food and human cases were subjected to antibiotic susceptibility testing, plasmid analysis, and serotyping. In 1984, the Seattle-King County Health Department prepared a report summarizing the results of the study. The 1984 study report found that *C. jejuni* was a more common cause of enteritis than *Salmonella*. Also, it concluded that *C. jejuni* "does appear to flow from chickens to man via consumption of poultry products" [4]. The report stated, "isolates from human cases and those from retail poultry had similar antibiotic susceptibility patterns, including prevalence of 29.7% and 32.8%, respectively, for tetracycline resistance, which was found to be plasmid-mediated" (*Ref. 4*, p. 3).

1988 Institute of Medicine (IOM) Report: "Human Health Risks with the Subtherapeutic Use of Penicillin or Tetracyclines in Animal Feed"

In 1987, FDA asked the IOM to conduct an independent review of the human health risks associated with the subtherapeutic use of penicillin and tetracycline in animal feed. IOM established a committee and directed it to perform "a quantitative risk assessment" of these human health consequences and to "assess the adequacy of the existing human health data and use such data to arrive at an estimate of risk" [5]. If quantification of human health risks was not possible due to inadequate data, the Committee was to evaluate the scientific information that had become available since the 1980 National Academy of Science report cited above.

The Committee developed a risk-analysis model, using data only on *Salmonella* infections that resulted in human death. However, the Committee was unable to find a substantial body of direct evidence demonstrating that the subtherapeutic use of penicillin or tetracycline in animal feed posed a human health hazard. Nonetheless, the Committee's 1988 report found a considerable body of indirect evidence implicating both subtherapeutic and therapeutic use of antimicrobials as a potential human health hazard. The Committee also strongly recommended further study of the issue.

1997 World Health Organization (WHO) Report, "The Medical Impact of Antimicrobial Use in Food Animals"

In October 1997, the WHO convened a meeting of experts to examine the question of whether the use of antimicrobials in livestock production, including through use in animal feed, contributes to the escalation of antimicrobial resistance in humans. The findings of the meeting, which were summarized in a report, included the conclusion that all uses of antimicrobials lead to the selection of resistant forms of bacteria. Furthermore, the report stated that "low-level, long-term exposure to antimicrobials may have greater selective potential than short-term, full-dose therapeutic use" [6]. The report found that the selection of resistant bacteria has adverse consequences for preventing and treating disease in humans, animals, and plants.

The WHO expert committee recommended that the use of antimicrobial drugs for growth promotion in animals be terminated if these drugs are also prescribed for use as anti-infective agents in human medicine or if they are known to induce cross-resistance to antimicrobials used for human medical therapy. The Committee also recommended the development of a systematic approach towards replacing growth-promoting antimicrobials with safer non-antimicrobial alternatives. The expert committee called for enhanced monitoring of resistance among isolates of enteric bacteria from food animals and food of animal origin. In addition, the Committee recommended managing risk at the primary production level through measures that promote the prudent use of antimicrobials, including enforcement of relevant laws pertaining to antimicrobial use, education for prescribers and producers, and requiring that use of antimicrobials for treatment of infections in animals be prescribed by veterinarians.

1999 National Research Council (NRC) Report: "The Use of Drugs in Food Animals – Benefits and Risks"

The Panel on Animal Health, Food Safety, and Public Health, jointly sponsored by the NRC's Board on Agriculture and IOM's Food and Nutrition Board, initiated a project to review the issues and relevant information regarding the use of drugs in food-producing animals and to make recommendations about such use. The panel convened the Committee on Drug Use in Food Animals to examine the benefits and risks associated with drug use in food-producing animals and to prepare a report and make recommendations.

The Committee's 1999 report included a review of the issues related to antibiotic use in food-producing animals and provided a number of recommendations. The report recommended establishing national databases to support scientific process and policy development for the approval and use of antibiotics in food-producing animals. The report also recommended that FDA use interdisciplinary panels of experts so that "further development and use of antibiotics in both human and animal medicine have oversight by an interdisciplinary panel of experts composed of representatives of the veterinary and animal health industry, the human medicine community, consumer advocacy groups, the animal production industry, and the regulatory agencies" [7].

1999 United States Government Accountability Office (GAO) Report – "Food Safety: The Agricultural Use of Antibiotics and Its Implications for Human Health"

In response to a request from Congress, the GAO initiated a study in May 1998 to examine: "1) how antibiotics are used in agriculture and the implications of that use for human health; 2) federal roles and responsibilities for overseeing the use of antibiotics in agriculture; and 3) issues surrounding the debate over whether to further regulate or restrict the use of antibiotics in agriculture" [8].

In its study report, dated April 1999, GAO concluded that although research has linked the use of antibiotics in agriculture to the emergence of resistant foodborne pathogens, "there are no current comprehensive estimates of the extent to which antibiotic-resistance strains have resulted in illness and deaths" [8]. GAO concluded that the debate over whether antibiotic use should be restricted in agriculture centers on the risk antibiotics pose to human health relative to their benefits to agriculture. The GAO report recommended that "the departments of Agriculture and Health and Human Services work together to develop and implement a plan with specific goals, time frames and resources needed for determining the safe use of antibiotics in agriculture."

1999 European Commission Report, "Opinion of the Scientific Steering Committee on Antimicrobial Resistance"

Due to the public and animal health concerns associated with the increasing rate of antimicrobial resistance development, the European

Commission, Directorate-General XXIV, asked that organization's Scientific Steering Committee to "scientifically evaluate the current position regarding the prevalence and development of antimicrobial resistance, examine its implications for human and animal health, particularly with regard to the development and management of infections" [9].

The Committee's report concluded that actions should be taken promptly to reduce the overall use of antimicrobials. Four primary recommendations were forwarded: (1) antimicrobial drugs should be used prudently; (2) infections should be prevented and resistant organisms contained; (3) research for new modalities of prevention and treatment of infections should be undertaken; and (4) the effects of such interventions should be monitored and evaluated.

2000 World Health Organization (WHO) Expert Consultation: "WHO Global Principles for the Containment of Antimicrobial Resistance in Animals Intended for Food"

The Food and Agriculture Organization of the United Nations (FAO) and the World Organization for Animal Health (OIE) participated in the June 2000 WHO expert consultation, the purpose of which was to develop global principles for minimizing the negative public health impact associated with the use of antimicrobial agents in food-producing animals while providing for their safe and effective use in veterinary medicine [10].

The principles were part of a comprehensive WHO global strategy for the containment of antimicrobial resistance and provided a framework of recommendations to reduce the overuse and misuse of antimicrobials in food-producing animals for the protection of human health. The principles strengthened and endorsed earlier WHO recommendations such as the need to terminate the use of antimicrobial growth promoters pending comprehensive human health safety evaluations, the need to ensure that all antimicrobials for animal use are only supplied through authorized outlets (e.g., by veterinary prescription), and the need to establish surveillance systems on antimicrobial drug consumption.

2003 Report, "Joint FAO/OIE/WHO Expert Workshop on Non-Human Antimicrobial Usage and Antimicrobial Resistance: Scientific Assessment"

In December 2003, the Food and Agriculture Organization of the United Nations (FAO), the World Organization for Animal Health (OIE), and the World Health Organization (WHO) convened a workshop to "perform a scientific assessment of the antimicrobial resistance risks arising from non-human usage of antimicrobials and to formulate recommendations and options for future risk management actions to be considered by the Codex Alimentarius Commission (Codex) and OIE" [11].

The expert panel's findings from the workshop were documented in a report which contained a number of conclusions, including: 1) "there is clear evidence of adverse human health consequences due to resistant organisms resulting from non-human usage of antimicrobials;" 2) "the amount and pattern of non-human usage of antimicrobials impact the occurrence of resistant bacteria in animals and on food commodities and thereby human exposure to these resistant bacteria;" 3) "the foodborne route is the major transmission pathway for resistant bacteria and resistance genes from food animals to humans, but other routes of transmission exist;" and 4) the "consequences of antimicrobial resistance are particularly severe when pathogens are resistant to antimicrobials critically important in humans" [11.]

The expert panel recommended that WHO appoint a group of experts to define which antimicrobials are considered critically important in humans. In addition, the panel commented on the need to further develop risk assessment approaches that adequately address the broad range of potential human health impacts and encouraged OIE to continue its work on risk analysis in coordination with FAO and WHO. Finally, the panel recommended that Codex collaborate with OIE to define a more efficient risk management system for addressing the risks.

2003 Institute of Medicine (IOM) Report, "Microbial Threats to Health: Emergence, Detection and Response"

The Committee on Emerging Microbial Threats to Health in the 21st Century was charged by the IOM to "review the current state of knowledge on the emergence of infectious diseases; assess the capacity of the United States to detect and respond to microbial threats to public health; and identify potential challenges and opportunities for public health actions, both global and domestic, to strengthen capabilities in prevention, detection, and response" [12].

The Committee's report discussed thirteen factors[4] that account for the emergence of new or enhanced microbial threats. The report noted "the convergence of any number of factors can create an environment where infectious diseases can emerge..." [12]. In addition, the Committee provided a number of recommended actions for responding to the increasing infectious disease rates prompted by these emergence factors. One of the recommendations was to "more finely target the use of antimicrobials" including expanding efforts to decrease the inappropriate use of antimicrobials in human medicine [12]. In addition, the committee recommended that "FDA ban the use of antimicrobials for growth promotion in animals if those classes of antimicrobials are also used in humans" [12].

2004 Report, "Second Joint FAO/OIE/WHO Expert Workshop on Non-Human Antimicrobial Usage and Antimicrobial Resistance: Management Options"

As summarized above, a preliminary scientific assessment of the antimicrobial resistance risks arising from non-human usage of antimicrobials was conducted by the first Joint Expert Workshop on Non-Human Antimicrobial Usage in December 2003 in Geneva [13]. The outcome of the first workshop, plus other relevant information, formed the basis for consideration by this second workshop. The report of this second workshop included suggestions to Codex, FAO, WHO, and OIE for moving forward on the issue.

Some of the key conclusions and recommendations in the report included: 1) the risks associated with non-human antimicrobial use and antimicrobial resistance should be part of human safety assessments for regulatory decisions relating to veterinary antimicrobials, 2) the concept of "critically-important" classes of antimicrobials for humans should be developed by WHO, 3) good agricultural practices can reduce the necessity for antimicrobials, 4) there is a need for capacity building and networking to help implement antimicrobial resistance surveillance systems in various countries, and 5) a Codex/OIE Task Force should be established to develop risk management options for antimicrobial resistance related to non-human use of antimicrobials.

2004 United States Government Accountability Office (GAO) Report – "Antibiotic Resistance: Federal Agencies Need to Better Focus Efforts to Address Risks to Humans from Antibiotic Use in Animals"

In response to a request from Congress, GAO initiated a study in May 2003 to "examine 1) scientific evidence on the transference of antibiotic resistance from animals to humans and extent of potential harm to human health, 2) agencies' efforts to assess and address these risks, 3) the types of data needed to support research on these risks and extent to which the agencies collect these data, 4) use of antibiotics in animals in the United States compared with its key agricultural trading partners and competitors, and 5) information on how use has affected trade" [14].

In its study report, dated April 2004, GAO concluded that antibiotic-resistant bacteria have been transferred from animals to humans. GAO also stated that many of the studies reviewed as part of GAO's research found that this transference from animals to humans poses significant risks for human health. According to GAO's findings, studies have shown two types of evidence related to the transfer of antibiotic-resistant bacteria from animals to humans. First, some studies have provided evidence of associations between changes in antibiotic use in animals and resistance to antibiotics in human bacteria. For example, researchers have found that antibiotic-resistant *Escherichia coli* (*E. coli*) and *Campylobacter* increased in humans as use of the antibiotics increased in animals.

Second, GAO concluded that studies that have examined the genetic makeup of the bacteria have provided stronger scientific evidence that antibiotic-resistant *Campylobacter* and *Salmonella* bacteria are transferred from animals to humans. In those studies, strains of antibiotic-resistant bacteria infecting humans were indistinguishable from those found in animals, leading researchers to conclude that the animals were the source of human infection.

The GAO report noted that researchers disagree about the extent of the human health risk caused by this transference. According to the report, "many researchers contend that antibiotic use in animals poses significant risk for human health." The GAO report also noted that "a small number of studies contend that the health risks of the transference are minimal" [14].

GAO recommended that "the Commissioner of FDA expedite FDA's risk assessments of the antibiotics used in animals that the agency has identified as critically important to human health to determine if action is necessary to restrict or prohibit animal uses in order to safeguard human health" (*Ref. 14*, p. 48). GAO also recommended that the Secretaries of Agriculture and of Health and Human Services "jointly develop and implement a plan for collecting data on antibiotic use in animals..." [14].

The Department of Health and Human Services (HHS) reviewed and subsequently responded to the 2004 GAO Report on Antibiotic Resistance. In its response, HHS cited 11 additional supporting studies not included in the GAO report (See End Note)[i], and provided the following comments:

"The draft report presents or refers to significant and growing evidence demonstrating the human health consequences of drug resistant infections related to antibiotic use in agriculture." "These [11 additional] studies, along with those cited in the GAO report, all demonstrate a relationship between the use of antimicrobials in food-producing animals, antibiotic resistance in humans, and adverse human health consequences as a result. We believe that there is a preponderance of evidence that the use of antimicrobials in food-producing animals has adverse human consequences." "There is little evidence to the contrary."

2005 Codex Alimentarius Commission (Codex), "Code of Practice to Minimize and Contain Antimicrobial Resistance" (Code of Practice)

The Code of Practice provides guidance for the responsible and prudent use of antimicrobials in food-producing animals [15]. Its objectives are to minimize adverse impacts on public health associated with the use of antimicrobial drugs in food-producing animals.

The Code of Practice makes a number of recommendations regarding the responsible use of antimicrobials in food-producing animals. For example, the document recommends that responsible use 1) should be controlled by the veterinary profession or other parties with the requisite expertise, and 2) does not include the use for growth promotion of veterinary antimicrobial drugs that belong to or are able to cause cross-resistance to classes of antimicrobial agents used in humans (or submitted for approval for use in humans) in the absence of an appropriate risk analysis.

2006 Antimicrobial Resistance: Implications for the Food System, Comprehensive Reviews in Food Science and Food Safety

This report was conducted under the auspices of the Institute of Food Technologists and the IFT foundation [16]. The panelists found the extent to which antibiotic use in food animals produces clinically important antibiotic resistant infections in humans is unknown. However, they do state in their recommendations that "In veterinary medicine and production agriculture implementation of various management strategies (such as responsible use guidelines, quality assurance programs, and antibiotic alternatives), coupled with government regulations, should decrease opportunities for the selection of antibiotic resistant microorganisms." Specifically, they stated "Always practice prudent use of antimicrobials to limit resistance selection and to maintain maximal benefit of antimicrobials in the future."

2009 American Academy of Microbiology. Antibiotic Resistance: An Ecological Perspective on an Old Problem

This report emphasizes the ecological fact that antibiotic resistance is a natural phenomenon that cannot be eliminated [17]. The practical approach is to find effective ways to cope with antibiotic resistant bacteria harmful to humans and animals and to control the development of new types of resistance. Controlling antibiotic-resistant bacteria and subsequent infections requires vigilance on many fronts. The prudent and responsible use of antibiotics and the elimination of unnecessary use (e.g., viral infections; unnecessary, prolonged treatment) are noted as mandatory steps to an appropriate public health strategy to limit infections by resistant organisms.

2011 WHO Report: Tackling Antibiotic Resistance from a Food Safety Perspective in Europe

This report follows a long series of WHO reports addressing antibiotic resistance in the food chain [18]. The WHO continues to highlight the urgent need for action in remediating antibiotic resistance through a holistic, intersectoral, and multifaceted approach that includes all efforts to reduce unnecessary use of antibiotics, including those uses in food production. Specific regulatory strategies include: 1) eliminating the use of antibiotics as growth promoters in food animals; 2) requiring that antibiotics be administered to animals only when prescribed by a veterinarian; and 3) requiring the antibiotics identified as critically important in human medicine - especially fluoroquinolones and third- and fourth-generation cephalosporins - only be used in food animals when their use is justified.

Brief Summary of Recent Peer-Reviewed Scientific Literature

2008. Applied and Environmental Microbiology. Longitudinal study of antimicrobial resistance among *Escherichia coli* isolates from integrated multisite cohorts of humans and swine. Alali et al.

This study longitudinally examined the relationship between antimicrobial resistant *E. coli* from human wastewater and swine fecal samples and several risk factors including host species, production type, vocation (e.g., slaughter plant workers), and season. Authors reported that the higher levels of *E. coli* resistance in swine isolates as compared with human isolates was likely associated with either the past or current use of injectable antimicrobial agents (e.g., ceftiofur sodium) or the use of antimicrobial agents in feed (e.g., chlortetracycline) or water. Furthermore, slaughter plant workers were shown to be at higher risk of carrying multidrug-resistant *E. coli* than non-swine workers.

2008. Applied and Environmental Microbiology. Diversity and Distribution of Commensal Fecal Escherichia Coli Bacteria in Beef Cattle Administered Selected Subtherapeutic Antimicrobials in a Feedlot Setting. Sharma et al.

This study investigated the influence of administration of chlortetracycline alone or in combination with sulfamethazine on the development of resistance, dissemination of defined strain types, and prevalence of resistance determinants in feedlot cattle [20]. Shedding of tetracycline-resistant *E. coli* was higher in animals receiving both treatments. While tetracycline resistance was detected in cattle with no prior antimicrobial exposure, shedding of tetracycline-resistant *E. coli* was higher in animals subjected to either of the two treatments.

2008. Applied and Environmental Microbiology. Effect of Subtherapeutic Administration of Antibiotics on the Prevalence of Antibiotic-Resistant Escherichia Coli Bacteria in Feedlot Cattle. Alexander et al.

This study involved the collection of 3,300 fecal samples over a 314-day period from 300 feedlot steers receiving subtherapeutic levels of antibiotics [21]. Study findings indicated that administration of tetracycline in combination with sulfamethazine clearly increased the prevalence of tetracycline- and ampicillin-resistant *E. coli* in cattle and the numbers of resistant *E. coli* organisms shed.

2009. American Journal of Veterinary Research. A Metagenomic Approach for Determining Prevalence of Tetracycline Resistance Genes in the Fecal Flora of Conventionally Raised Feedlot Steers and Feedlot Steers Raised Without Antimicrobials. Harvey et al.

This study compared the prevalence of tetracycline-resistance genes in the fecal flora of conventionally raised feedlot steers and feedlot steers raised without antimicrobials [22]. Authors observed that the percentage of fecal samples with 11 tetracycline resistance genes was significantly higher for fecal samples from conventionally raised cattle (35/61 [57%]) than for fecal samples from antimicrobial-free cattle (16/61 [26%]).

2009. Foodborne Pathogens and Disease. Association Between Tetracycline Consumption and Tetracycline Resistance in Escherichia Coli from Healthy Danish Slaughter Pigs. Vieira et al.

The objective of this Danish study was to investigate the association between tetracycline-resistant *Escherichia coli* isolates from the intestinal tract of healthy pigs and patterns of tetracycline consumption in the herds of origin, together with other risk factors [23]. The study showed that the larger the time since the last administration of tetracycline, the lower the likelihood of isolating a resistant *E. coli.*

2009. Preventive Veterinary Medicine. Associations Between Reported On-Farm Antimicrobial Use Practices and Observed Antimicrobial Resistance in Generic Fecal Escherichia Coli Isolated from Alberta Finishing Swine Farms. Varga et al.

This study used statistical models to evaluate the associations between various antimicrobial use practices and resistance to antimicrobials among generic fecal Escherichia coli isolated from Alberta finishing swine [24]. In-feed antimicrobial use was significantly associated with an increased risk of resistance to ampicillin, chloramphenicol, streptomycin, and sulfisoxazole in *E. coli* isolates. Chlortetracycline use in grower rations was associated with ampicillin and tetracycline resistance.

2010. International Journal of Food Microbiology. Farm-to-Fork Characterization of Escherichia Coli Associated with Feedlot Cattle with A Known History Of Antimicrobial Use. Alexander et al.

This study investigated antimicrobial-resistant *Escherichia coli* isolated from cattle fed diets containing chlortetracycline plus sulfamethazine (AS700) [25]. Compared to the control, in which no feed antibiotics were administered, the prevalence of ampicillin-resistant and tetracycline-resistant *E. coli* was three- and four-fold greater in feces from treated animals respectively, but was similar between treatments for animal hide samples.

2011. Environmental Health Perspectives. Lower Prevalence of Antibiotic-Resistant Enterococci on U.S. Conventional Poultry Farms That Transitioned to Organic Practices. Sapkota et al.

This study compared antimicrobial resistance in enterococci recovered from conventional poultry farms using antibiotics with farms that transitioned to antibiotic-free production practices and had just received organic certification [26]. Over 40% of *Enterococcus faecalis* isolates from conventional poultry houses were multidrug resistant, compared with 10% of isolates from newly organic poultry houses. In addition, 84% of *Enterococcus faecium* isolates from conventional poultry houses were multidrug resistant, compared with 17% of isolates from newly organic poultry houses.

2011. Foodborne Pathogens and Disease. Association Between Antimicrobial Resistance in Escherichia Coli Isolates from Food Animals and Blood Stream Isolates from Humans in Europe: An Ecological Study. Vieira et al.

The authors analyzed the correlation between the prevalence of antimicrobial resistance in *E. coli* isolates from blood stream infections in humans and in *E. coli* isolates from poultry, pigs, and cattle in 11 countries between 2005 and 2008 [27]. Resistance against multiple drugs in *E. coli* isolates from food animals (especially poultry and pigs) was highly correlated with resistance in isolates from humans.

2011. BMC Microbiology. Distribution and Characterization of Ampicillin- and Tetracycline-Resistant Escherichia Coli from Feedlot Cattle Fed Subtherapeutic Antimicrobials. Mirzaagha et al.

Authors characterized E. coli isolates recovered from cattle that either received no dietary antimicrobials or were intermittently administered subtherapeutic levels of chlortetracycline, chlortetracycline and sulfamethazine (SMX), or virginiamycin over a 9- month feeding period [28]. This study showed that strains exhibited multidrug resistance to SMX and chloramphenicol (a drug not in the antibiotic regimen) more frequently when obtained from steers fed chlortetracycline plus sulfamethazine than from cattle treated with either chlortetracycline alone or with virginiamycin. Results further suggested that the administration of chlortetracycline, even in the absence of SMX, can lead to the emergence of resistance to SMX, as well as other antibiotics, including ampicillin and chloramphenicol.

2012. Proceedings of the National Academy of Sciences. In-Feed Antibiotic Effects on the Swine Intestinal Microbiome. Looft et al.

This study involved pigs raised in a highly controlled environment, with one group of littermates receiving a diet containing a growth-enhancing antibiotic combination product [chlortetracycline, sulfamethazine, and penicillin (known as ASP250)] and the other receiving the same diet without the antibiotics [29]. Even a low, short-term (14-day) dose of in-feed antibiotics increased the prevalence and diversity of antibiotic resistance genes, including resistance to antibiotics not administered in the study, and increased the prevalence of *E. coli*.

IV. Strategies for Controlling Antimicrobial Resistance Are Needed

As summarized above in Section III, the public health concerns associated with the use of medically important antimicrobial drugs in food-producing animals have been the subject of scientific interest for the past 40 years. FDA has considered all available information and believes that the weight of scientific evidence supports the recommendations outlined in this guidance document.

To effectively respond to the public health concerns associated with antimicrobial resistance, FDA believes it is important to broadly consider how antimicrobial drugs are being used. The scientific community generally agrees that antimicrobial drug use is a key driver for the emergence of antimicrobial-resistant bacteria. It is imperative that strategies for controlling antimicrobial resistance include a consideration of how antimicrobial drugs are being used and measures to address those uses that are injudicious in nature.

V. Current Regulatory Framework

FDA considers the issue of antimicrobial resistance as part of its human food safety review related to new animal drugs used in food-producing animals. FDA considers an antimicrobial new animal drug to be "safe" if the agency concludes that there is "reasonable certainty of no harm to human health" from the proposed use of the drug in food-producing animals. This standard applies to safety evaluations completed prior to new animal drug approvals, as well as to those completed for drugs after approval. If this safety standard is not met before approval, the drug cannot be approved. If safety issues arise after approval, the Federal Food, Drug, and Cosmetic Act (the Act) provides grounds for withdrawal of approval of new animal drug applications for safety reasons. For example, section 512(e)(1)(B) of the Act provides for withdrawal of new animal drug application approvals when new evidence, along with evidence contained in the application, shows that the drug is not shown to be safe under the approved conditions of use. Under this provision, if FDA initiates a withdrawal action, it must produce evidence to show that there is a reasonable basis from which serious questions may be inferred about the ultimate safety of the drug and any substance that may be formed in or on food as a result of use of such drug under approved conditions. Once the agency meets this initial burden, the burden then shifts to the sponsor to demonstrate the safety of the drug (Docket no. 00N-1571, at p. 5, Mar. 16, 2004).

In 2003, FDA implemented new policies for evaluating antimicrobial resistance associated with use of antimicrobial new animal drugs in food-producing animals through the issuance of Guidance for Industry (GFI) #152, "Evaluating the Safety of Antimicrobial New Animal Drugs with Regard to their Microbiological Effects on Bacteria of Human Health Concern" (http://www.fda.gov/downloads/AnimalVeterinary/GuidanceComplianceEnforcement/GuidanceforIndustry/UCM052519.pdf). This guidance document describes a risk-based assessment process for evaluating antimicrobial resistance associated with the use of antimicrobial new animal drugs in food-producing animals. The guidance also recommends measures for mitigating such risk.

In general, FDA's GFI #152 is premised on the concept that increasing the exposure of bacterial populations to antimicrobial drugs increases the risk of generating resistance to those antimicrobial drugs. Pursuant to this principle, the administration of medically important antimicrobial drugs to entire herds or flocks of food-producing animals (e.g., for production purposes) would represent a use that poses a qualitatively higher risk to public health than the administration of such drugs to individual animals or targeted groups of animals (e.g., to prevent, control, or treat specific diseases). In addition to factors that impact the potential extent of use of the drug, the guidance also considers such factors as the properties of the drug in question including mechanism of action and mechanism of resistance, the prevalence of zoonotic foodborne bacteria in the food-producing animal species for which the drug is intended, and the importance of the drug in question as a therapy in humans. Risk mitigating factors that are considered include such limitations as restricting use of the drug to use by or on the order of a veterinarian.

Although FDA developed GFI #152 primarily to assess antimicrobial resistance risks as part of the new animal drug approval process, the underlying concept described above is also applicable to safety evaluations conducted for previously-approved antimicrobial new animal drugs. Therefore, FDA considers this same concept when it conducts safety evaluations for currently approved antimicrobial drugs, including those approved for use in animal feed.

From a practical standpoint, however, some significant differences exist between applying the GFI #152 risk assessment approach to the pre-approval process and applying it to safety reviews of currently-approved products. On the pre-approval side, the GFI #152 assessment process, including the various risk mitigation measures described, is taken into consideration by drug sponsors upstream in the drug development process and, in effect, steers product development in a direction that is most consistent with the guidance. On the post-approval side, FDA may examine certain currently-approved products to determine whether such products appear consistent with GFI #152. However, initiating action to withdraw an approved new animal drug application (NADA), in whole or in part, based on the results of a post-approval safety review would require the agency to make the showing required under section 512(e)(1) of the Act.

Alternatively, concerns associated with approved NADAs can sometimes be addressed through more informal processes. For example, in certain cases FDA has worked collaboratively with the sponsor of an NADA to address concerns raised regarding their product and has initiated steps to permit the sponsor to voluntarily withdraw part or all of the NADA or to revise the product labeling to address the concern. This alternative pathway can in some cases be an effective and expedient mechanism for resolving issues associated with an NADA.

VI. Status of FDA's Current Activities

In general, the antimicrobial new animal drug applications that FDA is addressing as part of its efforts to evaluate the public health concerns associated with the use of medically important antimicrobial drugs in food-producing animals can be divided into two broad categories: 1) those NADAs submitted after the issuance of GFI #152 in 2003 and for which FDA is assessing the microbiological safety of the new animal drug on a pre-approval basis using the principles outlined in GFI #152; and 2) those NADAs approved before the final version of GFI#152 was issued in 2003. In regard to the first category, FDA believes the approach outlined in GFI #152 for evaluating microbiological safety as part of the drug approval process has been very effective. As noted above, that assessment process and the associated risk mitigation measures are usually taken into consideration by industry during the drug development process. Thus, products that ultimately move forward toward approval are those products that include use conditions that are consistent with the guidance and are intended to minimize the extent to which product use would contribute to resistance development.

FDA believes the approach outlined in GFI #152 is scientifically sound and is protective of the public health. FDA recognizes that the list of drugs in Appendix A is not static and should be periodically reassessed and updated as necessary. Such reassessment is necessary to take into consideration such factors as the development of new antimicrobials for human therapy, the emergence of diseases in humans, or changes in prescribing practices in the United States. FDA will update Appendix A, as necessary, through a separate process that will also be subject to public comment.

The second category of products are those antimicrobial NADAs that were approved prior to the implementation of GFI #152. Some of the products in this category include products that were approved for use in food-producing animals more than 30 years ago. Of particular concern, as discussed in section IV, are those products that are approved for use in animal feed for production or growth-enhancing purposes. Although these products are FDA-approved, their approval occurred prior to implementation of current processes for assessing safety with respect to antimicrobial resistance. Furthermore, the scientific understanding regarding antimicrobial resistance has advanced significantly over this time frame and, as discussed earlier in this document, a number of scientific reports have raised public health concerns regarding the use of medically important antimicrobials in food-producing animals.

As a result, FDA is examining available information regarding medically important antimicrobial drugs currently approved for use in food-producing animals and considering potential steps for agency action.

VII. Recommended Principles Regarding Judicious Use in Animals

The continued availability of effective antimicrobial drugs is critically important for combating infectious disease in both humans and animals. This includes the continued availability of feed and water uses of such drugs for managing disease in animal agriculture. Therefore, it is in the interest of both human and animal health that we take a more proactive approach to considering how antimicrobial drugs are being used, and take steps to assure that such uses are appropriate and necessary for maintaining the health of humans and animals. Using medically important antimicrobial drugs as judiciously as possible is key to minimizing resistance development and preserving the effectiveness of these drugs as therapies for humans and animals. Although FDA applauds the efforts to date by various veterinary and animal producer organizations to institute guidelines for the judicious use of antimicrobial drugs, the agency believes additional, voluntary steps are needed.

To further address this public and animal health concern, FDA is recommending two additional principles about the appropriate or judicious use of medically important antimicrobial drugs in food-producing animals. These principles are consistent with the recommendations of a number of recent scientific panels or committees referenced earlier in this document including the 1997, 2000, and 2011 reports of the WHO, the 2003 IOM Report, and the 2005 Codex Code of Practice.

FDA recognizes the need to collaborate with the animal health and animal producer communities on strategies for minimizing animal health impacts or industry disruption that may be associated with the implementation of changes by animal drug sponsors to voluntarily align the use conditions of affected drug products with the principles outlined below. Furthermore, FDA intends to consult with the United States Department of Agriculture (USDA) on implementation strategies, including the development of a framework for veterinary oversight and consultation requirements. FDA is committed to assuring that the public health is protected while also assuring that the health needs of animals are addressed.

Principle 1: The use of medically important antimicrobial drugs in food-producing animals should be limited to those uses that are considered necessary for assuring animal health.

In light of the risk that antimicrobial resistance poses to public health, FDA believes the use of medically important antimicrobial drugs in food-producing animals for production purposes (e.g., to promote growth or improve feed efficiency) represents an injudicious use of these important drugs. Production uses are not directed at any specifically identified disease, but rather are expressly indicated and used for the purpose of enhancing the production of animal-derived products. In contrast, FDA considers uses that are associated with the treatment, control, or prevention[5] of specific diseases, including administration through feed or water, to be uses that are necessary for assuring the health of food-producing animals.

Some may have concerns that the use of medically important antimicrobial drugs in food-producing animals for disease prevention purposes is not an appropriate or judicious use. However, FDA believes that some indications for prevention use are necessary and judicious as long as such use includes professional veterinary involvement. Veterinary involvement in the decision-making process associated with the use of medically important antimicrobial drugs is an important aspect of assuring appropriate use, including judicious prevention use. When determining the appropriateness of a prevention use, veterinarians consider several important factors such as determining the medical rationale for such use, and that such use is appropriately targeted at a specific etiologic agent and appropriately timed relative to the disease. For example, if a veterinarian determines, based on the client's production practices and herd health history, that cattle being transported or otherwise stressed are more likely to develop a certain bacterial infection, preventively treating these cattle with an antimicrobial approved for prevention of that bacterial infection would be considered a judicious use. Another example would be the prevention of necrotic enteritis in broiler chickens. In this case, the prevention use of an antimicrobial is important to manage this disease in certain flocks in the face of concurrent coccidiosis, a significant parasitic disease in chickens. On the other hand, FDA would not consider the administration of a drug to apparently healthy animals in the absence of any information that such animals were at risk of a specific disease to be a judicious use. The decision to use a specific drug or combination drug is generally based on factors that veterinarians are uniquely qualified to consider, including the mode of antibacterial action, drug distribution in specific tissues, and the duration of effective drug levels at the site of infection.

Principle 2: The use of medically important antimicrobial drugs in food-producing animals should be limited to those uses that include veterinary oversight or consultation.

Most of the feed-use antimicrobial drugs are currently approved for over-the-counter use in food-producing animals for purposes that include the treatment, control, and prevention of disease as well as for production purposes (i.e., for growth promotion uses such as increased rate of weight gain). In addition to instituting voluntary measures that would limit use of medically important antimicrobial drugs in food-producing animals to uses that are considered necessary to assure the animals' health, FDA also believes it is important to phase-in the voluntary practice of including veterinary oversight or consultation in the use of these drugs. As noted above, FDA believes that this practice is an important mechanism for helping to assure appropriate use. Veterinarians can play a critical role in the diagnosis of disease and in the decision-making process related to instituting measures to treat, control, or prevent disease. FDA recognizes that the nature of veterinary involvement can vary due to numerous factors such as geographic location and animal production setting. In fact, there are limited numbers of large animal veterinarians, which can make consultation or oversight challenging in certain situations. For example, some animal disease events require immediate attention. In some cases, veterinarians may be directly diagnosing and administering therapies, while in other cases they are visiting and consulting with producers periodically to establish customized disease management protocols for that producer's herd or flock. Of key importance to FDA is the fact that, in both of these cases, the veterinarian is involved in the decision-making process regarding antimicrobial drug use. FDA recognizes that increasing veterinary involvement in the use of antimicrobial drugs has significant practical implications for animal producers, veterinary practitioners, and the veterinary profession as whole. Therefore, FDA is particularly interested in receiving comments on strategies for effectively promoting the voluntary adoption of such a change.

CONCLUSION

In order to minimize the development of antimicrobial resistance, FDA believes that it is important to ensure the judicious use of medically important antimicrobial drugs in animal agriculture. We recommend several steps to accomplish this including voluntary measures that would limit medically important antimicrobial drugs to uses in food-producing animals that are considered necessary for assuring animal health and that include veterinary oversight or consultation. Such limitations would reduce overall medically important antimicrobial drug use levels, thereby reducing antimicrobial resistance selection pressure, while still maintaining the availability of these drugs for appropriate use.

REFERENCES

[1] 1969 Report of the Joint Committee on the Use of Antibiotics in Animal Husbandry and Veterinary Medicine.

[2] 1970 FDA Task Force Report, "The Use of Antibiotics in Animal Feed."
[3] 1980 National Academy of Sciences Report, "The Effects on Human Health of Subtherapeutic Use of Antimicrobial Drugs in Animal Feeds."
[4] 1984 Seattle-King County Study: "Surveillance of the Flow of *Salmonella* and *Campylobacter* in a Community."
[5] 1988 Institute of Medicine (IOM) Report: "Human Health Risks with the Subtherapeutic Use of Penicillin or Tetracyclines in Animal Feed."
[6] 1997 World Health Organization (WHO) Report, "The Medical Impact of Antimicrobial Use in Food Animals." http://whqlibdoc.who.int/hq/1997/WHO_EMC_ZOO_97.4.pdf.
[7] 1999 National Research Council (NRC) Report: "The Use of Drugs in Food Animals – Benefits and Risks."
[8] 1999 United States Government Accountability Office (GAO) Report – "Food Safety: The Agricultural Use of Antibiotics and Its Implications for Human Health." http://www.gao.gov/archive/1999/rc99074.pdf.
[9] 1999 European Commission Report, "Opinion of the Scientific Steering Committee on Antimicrobial Resistance." http://ec.europa.eu/food/fs/sc/ssc/out50 en.pdf.
[10] 2000 World Health Organization (WHO) Expert Consultation: "WHO Global Principles for the Containment of Antimicrobial Resistance in Animals Intended for Food." http://whqlibdoc.who.int/hq/2000/WHO CDS CSR APH 2000.4.pdf.
[11] 2003 Report, "Joint FAO/OIE/WHO Expert Workshop on Non-Human Antimicrobial Usage and Antimicrobial Resistance: Scientific assessment." http://www.who.int/ foodsafety/publications/micro/en/amr.pdf.
[12] 2003 Institute of Medicine (IOM) Report, "Microbial Threats to Health: Emergence, Detection and Response."
[13] 2004 Report, "Second Joint FAO/OIE/WHO Expert Workshop on Non-Human Antimicrobial Usage and Antimicrobial Resistance: Management options." http://www.oie.int/fileadmin/Home/eng/Conferences_Events/docs/pdf/WHO-CDSCPE-ZFK-2004.8.pdf.
[14] 2004 United States Government Accountability Office (GAO) Report – "Antibiotic Resistance: Federal Agencies Need to Better Focus Efforts to Address Risks to Humans from Antibiotic Use in Animals." http://www.gao.gov/new.items/d04490.pdf.
[15] 2005 Codex Alimentarius Commission (Codex), "Code of Practice to Minimize and Contain Antimicrobial Resistance." http://www.codex alimentarius.net/download/standards/10213/CXP 061e.pdf.

[16] 2006 Antimicrobial Resistance: Implications for the Food System, Comprehensive Reviews in Food Science and Food Safety, Vol. 5, 2006.

[17] 2009. American Academy of Microbiology. Antibiotic Resistance: An Ecological Perspective on an Old Problem. 1752 N Street, NW Washington, DC 20036 http://www.asm.org.

[18] 2011. Tackling antibiotic resistance from a food safety perspective in Europe. World Health Organization (WHO), Regional Office for Europe Scherfigsvej 8, DK-2100 Copenhagen Ø, Denmark. http://www.euro.who.int/data/assets/pdffile/0005/ 136454/e94889.pdf.

[19] 2008. Longitudinal study of antimicrobial resistance among *Escherichia coli* isolates from integrated multisite cohorts of humans and swine. Alali WQ, Scott HM, Harvey RB, Norby B, Lawhorn DB, Pillai SD. *Appl. Environ. Microbiol.* 74(12):3672-81.

[20] 2008. Diversity and distribution of commensal fecal *Escherichia coli* bacteria in beef cattle administered selected subtherapeutic antimicrobials in a feedlot setting. Sharma R, Munns K, Alexander T, Entz T, Mirzaagha P, Yanke LJ, Mulvey M, Topp E, McAllister T. *Appl. Environ. Microbiol.*;74(20):6178-86.

[21] 2008. Effect of subtherapeutic administration of antibiotics on the prevalence of antibiotic-resistant *Escherichia coli* bacteria in feedlot cattle. Alexander, T.W., L.J. Yanke, E. Topp, M.E. Olson, R.R. Read, D.W. Morck, and T.A. McAllister. *Applied and Environmental Microbiology*. 74:4405-4416.

[22] 2009. A metagenomic approach for determining prevalence of tetracycline resistance genes in the fecal flora of conventionally raised feedlot steers and feedlot steers raised without antimicrobials. Harvey, R., J. Funk, T.E. Wittum, and A.E. Hoet. *American Journal of Veterinary Research.* 70:198-202.

[23] 2009. Association between tetracycline consumption and tetracycline resistance in *Escherichia coli* from healthy Danish slaughter pigs. Vieira, A.R., H. Houe, H.C. Wegener, D.M. Lo Fo Wong, and H.D. Emborg. *Foodborne Pathogens and Disease*. 6:99-109.

[24] 2009. Associations between reported on-farm antimicrobial use practices and observed antimicrobial resistance in generic fecal *Escherichia coli* isolated from Alberta finishing swine farms. Varga C., A. Rajic, M.E. McFall, R.J. Reid-Smith, A.E. Deckert, S.L. Checkley, and S.A. McEwen. *Preventive Veterinary Medicine.* 88:185-192.

[25] 2010. Farm-to-fork characterization of *Escherichia coli* associated with feedlot cattle with a known history of antimicrobial use. Alexander,

T.W., G.D. Inglis, L.J. Yanke, E. Topp, R.R. Read, T. Reuter, and T.A. McAllister. *International Journal of Food Microbiology*. 137:40-48.

[26] 2011. Lower prevalence of antibiotic-resistant Enterococci on U.S. conventional poultry farms that transitioned to organic practices. Sapkota AR, Hulet RM, Zhang G, McDermott P, Kinney EL, Schwab KJ, Joseph SW. *Environ. Health Perspect.* 119(11):1622-8.

[27] 2011. Association between antimicrobial resistance in *Escherichia coli* isolates from food animals and blood stream isolates from humans in Europe: an ecological study. Foodborne Pathogens and Disease. Vieira, A.R., P. Collignon, F.M. Aarestrup, S.A. McEwen, R.S. Hendriksen, T. Hald, and H.C. Wegener. 8:1295-1301.

[28] 2011. Distribution and characterization of ampicillin- and tetracycline-resistant *Escherichia coli* from feedlot cattle fed subtherapeutic antimicrobials. Mirzaagha P, Louie M, Sharma R, Yanke LJ, Topp E, McAllister TA. *BMC Microbiol.* 19;11:78.

[29] 2012. In-feed antibiotic effects on the swine intestinal microbiome. Looft, T., T.A. Johnson, H.K. Allen, D.O. Bayles, D.P. Alt, R.D. Stedtfeld, W.J. Sul, T.M. Stedtfeld, B. Chai, J.R. Cole, S.A. Hashsham, J.M. Tiedje, and T.B. Stanton. *Proceedings of the National Academy of Sciences USA*. 109:1691-1696.

NOTE

Other studies referenced by the Department of Health and Human Services in response to 2004 United States Government Accountability Office (GAO) Report – "Antibiotic Resistance: Federal Agencies Need to Better Focus Efforts to Address Risks to Humans from Antibiotic Use in Animals":

Helms M, Vastrup P, Gerner-Smidt P, Mølbak K. Excess mortality associated with antimicrobial drug-resistant Salmonella Typhimurium. Emerg Infect Dis 2002;8:490-5.

Holmberg SD, Solomon SL, Blake PA. Health and economic impacts of antimicrobial resistance. Rev Infect Dis 1987; 9:1065-78.

Holmberg SD, Wells JG, Cohen ML. Animal-to-man transmission of antimicrobial-resistant Salmonella: investigations of U.S. outbreaks, 1971-1983. Science 1984;225:833-5.

Lee LA, Puhr ND, Maloney K, et al. Increase in antimicrobial-resistant Salmonella infections in the United States, 1989-1990. J Infect Dis 1994;170:128-34.

Martin L, Fyfe M, Doré K, et al. Increased burden of illness associated with antimicrobial-resistant Salmonella enterica serotype Typhimurium infections. J Infect Dis 2004;189:377-84.

Neimann J, Mølbak K, Engberg J, et al. Longer duration of illness among Campylobacter patients treated with fluoroquinolones. 11th International Workshop on Campylobacter, Helicobacter, and Related Organisms, 1-5 September, 2001. Freiburg, Germany.

Nelson JM, Smith KE, Vugia DJ, et al. Prolonged diarrhea due to ciprofloxacinresistant Campylobacter infections. J Infect Dis 2004; 190:1150-7.

Phillips I, Casewell M, Cox T, et al. Does the use of antibiotics in food animals pose a risk to human health? A critical review of published data. J Antimicrob Chemother 2004;53:28-52.

Smith KE, Besser JM, Hedberg CW, et al. Quinolone-resistant Campylobacter jejuni infections in Minnesota, 1992-1998. N Engl J Med 1999;340:1525-32.

Varma J, Mølbak K, Rossiter S, et al. Antimicrobial resistance in Salmonella is associated with increased hospitalization; NARMS 1996-2000. International Conference on Emerging Infectious Diseases. March 2002. Atlanta, GA.

Varma J, Mølbak K, Rossiter S, et al. Antimicrobial resistance in non-typhoidal Salmonella is associated with increased hospitalization and bloodstream infection-- United States, 1996-2000. 51st Annual EIS Conference. April 22-26, 2002. Atlanta, GA.

End Notes

[1] The term "medically important antimicrobial drugs" generally refers to antimicrobial drugs that are important for therapeutic use in humans.

[2] The term "antimicrobial" refers broadly to drugs with activity against a variety of microorganisms including bacteria, viruses, fungi, and parasites. Antimicrobial drugs that have specific activity against bacteria are referred to as antibacterial or antibiotic drugs. However, the broader term "antimicrobial," commonly used in reference to drugs with activity against bacteria, is used in this document interchangeably with the terms antibacterial or antibiotic. Antimicrobial resistance is the ability of bacteria or other microbes to resist the effects of a drug. Antimicrobial resistance, as it relates to bacterial

organisms, occurs when bacteria change in some way that reduces or eliminates the effectiveness of drugs, chemicals, or other agents designed to treat bacterial infections.

[3] Production uses are also referred to as "nontherapeutic" or "subtherapeutic" uses, terms that we believe lack sufficient clarity.

[4] The thirteen factors included 1) microbial adaptation and change, 2) human vulnerability, 3) climate and weather, 4) changing ecosystems, 5) economic development and land use, 6) human demographics and behavior, 7) technology and industry, 8) international travel and commerce, 9) breakdown of public health measures, 10) poverty and social inequality, 11) war and famine, 12) lack of political will, and 13) intent to harm.

[5] Disease prevention involves the administration of an antimicrobial drug to animals, none of which are exhibiting clinical signs of disease, in a situation where disease is likely to occur if the drug is not administered.

In: Antibiotic Use in U.S. Livestock Production ISBN: 978-1-63485-056-8
Editor: Karin Greer

Chapter 3

GUIDANCE FOR INDUSTRY: NEW ANIMAL DRUGS AND NEW ANIMAL DRUG COMBINATION PRODUCTS ADMINISTERED IN OR ON MEDICATED FEED OR DRINKING WATER OF FOOD-PRODUCING ANIMALS: RECOMMENDATIONS FOR DRUG SPONSORS FOR VOLUNTARILY ALIGNING PRODUCT USE CONDITIONS WITH GFI #209*

Food and Drug Administration

This guidance represents the Food and Drug Administration's (FDA's) current thinking on this topic. It does not create or confer any rights for or on any person and does not operate to bind FDA or the public. You can use an alternative approach if the approach satisfies the requirements of the applicable statutes and regulations. If you want to discuss an alternative approach, contact the FDA staff responsible for implementing this guidance. If you cannot identify the appropriate FDA staff, call the number listed on the previous page of this guidance.

---

* This is an edited, reformatted and augmented version of guidance document #213, issued by the U.S. Food and Drug Administration, Center for Veterinary Medicine, December 2013.

I. INTRODUCTION

This guidance is intended for sponsors of approved applications for new animal drugs and new animal drug combination products containing medically important antimicrobial new animal drugs for use in or on medicated feed or water of food-producing animals. The guidance contains information for sponsors of such new animal drugs and combination products to facilitate voluntary changes to the conditions of use for such new animal drugs and combination products consistent with FDA's recommendations included in the guidance document entitled "The Judicious Use of Medically Important Antimicrobial Drugs in Food-Producing Animals" (Judicious Use Guidance, GFI #209). In particular, the purpose of this guidance is to provide sponsors with specific recommendations on how to supplement their approved new animal drug applications to align with FDA's GFI #209.

FDA's guidance documents, including this guidance, do not establish legally enforceable responsibilities. Instead, guidances describe the FDA's current thinking on a topic and should be viewed only as recommendations, unless specific regulatory or statutory requirements are cited. The use of the word "should" in FDA's guidances means that something is suggested or recommended, but not required.

II. BACKGROUND

On April 11, 2012, FDA finalized a guidance document entitled "The Judicious Use of Medically Important Antimicrobial Drugs in Food-Producing Animals" (Judicious Use Guidance, GFI #209). That final guidance represents the Agency's current thinking regarding antimicrobial drugs that are medically important in human medicine and used in food-producing animals. Specifically, the final guidance discusses FDA's concerns regarding the development of antimicrobial resistance in human and animal bacterial pathogens when medically important antimicrobial drugs are used in food-producing animals in an injudicious manner. In addition, the Judicious Use Guidance provides two recommended principles regarding the appropriate or judicious use of medically important antimicrobial drugs:

1) Limit medically important antimicrobial drugs to uses in animals that are considered necessary for assuring animal health, and

2) Limit medically important antimicrobial drugs to uses in animals that include veterinary oversight or consultation.

As noted above, the purpose of this guidance is to provide sponsors with specific recommendations on how to voluntarily modify the use conditions of their medically important antimicrobial drug products to align with the above two principles. The voluntary process outlined in this guidance would help to phase out the use of medically important antimicrobial drugs for production purposes and phase in veterinary oversight of therapeutic uses of these drugs.

A. Therapeutic Uses that Help Assure the Health of Animals

As discussed in GFI #209, FDA believes that, in light of the risk that antimicrobial resistance poses to public health, the use of medically important antimicrobial drugs for production purposes in food-producing animals does not represent a judicious use of these drugs. Such uses are typically administered through the feed or water on a herd- or flock-wide basis and are currently approved for such uses as increasing rate of weight gain or improving feed efficiency.

Production uses are not directed at any specifically identified disease, but rather are expressly indicated and used for the purpose of enhancing the production of animal-derived products. FDA believes that production use indications such as "increased rate of weight gain" or "improved feed efficiency" are no longer appropriate for the approved conditions of use for medically important antimicrobial drugs. In contrast, FDA considers uses that are associated with the treatment, control, and prevention of specific diseases to be therapeutic uses that are necessary for assuring the health of food-producing animals.

B. Veterinary Oversight

New animal drugs and new animal drug combination products are approved with one of three types of marketing status: (1) over-the-counter (OTC), (2) veterinary prescription (Rx), or (3) veterinary feed directive (VFD). Products for which adequate directions for use can be written for use by lay persons are labeled for OTC marketing status. When adequate directions can not be written in a manner that enables a layperson to use a drug safely and for the purposes for which it is intended, the drug is restricted to use under veterinary oversight as an Rx or VFD product.

FDA believes it is important to include veterinary oversight in the use of antimicrobial new animal drugs to assure their appropriate and judicious use. Veterinarians play a critical role in the diagnosis of disease and in the decision-making process related to instituting measures to treat, control, or prevent disease. As discussed in more detail below, FDA believes that the judicious use of medically important antimicrobial new animal drugs in the feed or water of food-producing animals needs the scientific and clinical training of a licensed veterinarian.

III. Medically Important Antimicrobial Drugs

FDA uses the concepts set out in its Guidance for Industry (GFI) #152, "*Evaluating the Safety of Antimicrobial New Animal Drugs with Regard to their Microbiological Effects on Bacteria of Human Health Concern*," in reviewing the human food safety component of new animal drug applications for medically important antimicrobial new animal drugs for use in food-producing animals. Guidance for Industry #152 includes an appendix that ranks antimicrobial drugs into three tiers, "critically important," "highly important," or "important," in regard to their human medical importance. At this time, FDA considers all antimicrobial drugs listed in Appendix A to GFI #152 (Appendix A) to be "medically important" in the context of implementing the recommendations outlined in GFI #209 and further discussed in this guidance document (GFI #213). We believe that the policy in GFI #209 and GFI #213 applies to all three tiers of medically important antimicrobial drugs at this time because each tier (and thus all of the drugs listed in Appendix A) contains drugs that have been previously assessed through the public processes used to develop GFI#152 and determined to be important for treating bacterial infections in people.

FDA recognizes that the list of drugs in Appendix A is not static and should be periodically reassessed and updated as necessary. Such reassessment is necessary to take into consideration such factors as the development of new antimicrobials for human therapy, the emergence of diseases in humans, or changes in prescribing practices in the United States. FDA intends to update Appendix A, as necessary, through a separate process that will also be subject to public comment. However, because Appendix A identifies those antimicrobials that have been determined to be medically important to human medicine, FDA believes the existing Appendix A provides adequate clarity for purposes of moving forward with the recommendations outlined in GFI #209. Therefore, the current list of medically important antimicrobial drug classes that are the subject of this guidance includes: aminoglycosides, lincosamides, macrolides, penicillins, streptogramins, sulfonamides, and tetracyclines.

IV. Voluntary Adoption of Judicious Use Principles

As discussed in the following section, FDA intends to work with affected drug sponsors to help them to voluntarily implement the principles described above through modifications to the approved conditions of use of their new animal drug products. FDA believes a voluntary approach, conducted in a cooperative and timely manner, is the most effective approach to achieve the common goal of more judicious use of medically important antimicrobials in animal agriculture.

FDA recognizes that it is equally important that the Agency also work with the veterinary and animal producer communities, the end users of these products, to ensure that their concerns are taken into consideration as these changes are implemented. One issue of concern is the ability of producers, particularly those with smaller operations in remote locations, to have adequate access to veterinary services. Therefore, as steps are taken to phase in the voluntary changes discussed in this document, FDA is working collaboratively with United States Department of Agriculture (USDA) to engage the veterinary community and other stakeholders to explore strategic approaches (e.g., new models, pilot programs) to address this issue.

A. Voluntarily Phasing out Production Uses

FDA is concerned about the risk that antimicrobial resistance poses to public health from the use of medically important antimicrobial drugs in food-producing animals for production purposes. As a consequence of this concern, FDA will be working with affected drug sponsors who wish to voluntarily withdraw approved production uses of their medically important antimicrobial new animal drugs and combination new animal drug products. This guidance is intended to facilitate the voluntary process by providing useful information for sponsors intending to revise their approved labeling through a supplemental new animal drug application. In addition, as discussed later in this guidance, FDA is asking affected sponsors to notify the Agency within 3 months from the date of publication of this final guidance to inform us of their intentions to make these voluntary changes.

B. Need for Veterinary Oversight of Medically Important Antimicrobial Drugs Used in the Feed or Water of Food-Producing Animals

Prior to 1993, most antimicrobial drugs were approved for over-the-counter use in food-producing animals and many of these were administered through medicated feed or drinking water. At that time, the methods used by FDA to assess the microbial food safety aspects of new animal drug applications for antimicrobials intended for use in food-producing animals were not as rigorous as those used today, in part because less scientific data about the public health ramifications of antimicrobial resistance existed at that time. In addition, FDA's recommended approach for conducting pre-approval microbial food safety assessments has evolved over time as the quantity and quality of epidemiologic and other data bearing on antimicrobial resistance has improved. As a result, all antimicrobial new animal drugs for use in food-producing animals approved by CVM since 1993 have been labeled with Rx or VFD marketing status, with the exception of approvals of generic copies of existing OTC products and approvals of combination medicated feeds using existing OTC antimicrobial Type A medicated articles[1]. This shift to a marketing status requiring veterinary oversight was viewed as an important step to mitigate the microbial food safety risks of antimicrobial new animal drugs, particularly for those drugs considered to be medically important.

Based on the available scientific evidence concerning antimicrobial resistance, including information about resistance trends associated with the use of medically important antimicrobial drugs in food-producing animals, FDA believes that the judicious use of medically important antimicrobial drugs intended for use in food-producing animals should involve the scientific and clinical training of a licensed veterinarian. This is because judicious use involves accurately identifying bacterial disease that is present or likely to be present and selecting the suitable antimicrobial drug.

In the case of prevention, judicious use includes a consideration by the veterinarian of relevant factors for determining the risk of a specific bacterial disease and for determining whether the use of medically important antimicrobials for prevention purposes is appropriate in a particular situation. The decision by the veterinarian to use a specific approved drug or combination drug is based on factors such as the mode of antibacterial action, drug distribution in specific tissues, and the duration of effective drug levels at the site of infection. Other important factors veterinarians consider when determining the appropriateness of a preventive use include whether: (1) there is evidence of effectiveness, (2) such a preventive use is consistent with accepted veterinary practice, (3) the use is linked to a specific etiologic agent, (4) the use is appropriately targeted to animals at risk of developing a specific disease, and (5) no reasonable alternatives for intervention exist. Numerous risk factors have been documented to increase susceptibility to bacterial disease, including environmental factors (such as temperature extremes and inadequate ventilation), host factors (such as age, nutrition, genetics, immune status), and other factors (such as stress of animal transport). From FDA's standpoint, the administration of a drug to animals when a veterinarian determines that there is a risk of a specific disease, based on the presence of such risk factors, could be considered judicious prevention use. For example, if a veterinarian determines, based on the client's production practices and herd health history, that cattle being transported or otherwise stressed are more likely to develop a certain bacterial infection, preventively treating these cattle with an antimicrobial approved for prevention of that bacterial infection would be considered a judicious use. Another example would be the prevention of necrotic enteritis in broiler chickens. In this case, the preventive use of an antimicrobial approved for such use is important to manage this disease in certain flocks in the face of concurrent coccidiosis, a significant parasitic disease in chickens. On the other hand, FDA would not consider the administration of a drug to apparently healthy animals in the absence of any information that such animals were at risk of a specific disease to be judicious. FDA believes that veterinarians are uniquely qualified to determine which specific disease-causing microorganisms are likely to be present in a particular situation and to determine appropriately timed administration to prevent disease based on specific, known risk.

For these reasons, in FDA's 1999 proposed rule on veterinary feed directives (64 FR 35966; July 2, 1999), the Agency gave antimicrobial resistance as a key example of a reason it can be important for medicated feed to be administered under a veterinarian's supervision. FDA stated, "control of the usage of certain antimicrobials is critical to reducing unnecessary use of such drugs in animals and to slowing or preventing the development of bacterial resistance to antimicrobial drugs."

Accordingly, FDA recommends that affected drug sponsors voluntarily revise the conditions of use of their medically important antimicrobial new animal drugs and combination new animal drug products to reflect the need for the professional oversight of a licensed veterinarian. This would mean a change from OTC to VFD status for medicated feed products and from OTC to Rx status for medicated drinking water products. A proposed timeline for making such changes is discussed in more detail below. FDA acknowledges that in order to facilitate the OTC to VFD change in marketing status, existing requirements related to the distribution and use of VFD drugs must be updated and streamlined. Therefore, concurrent with the development of this guidance, FDA is actively pursuing revisions to the VFD regulations (in 21 CFR part 558) through the rulemaking process. Some of the key changes being considered include better alignment between the criteria for appropriate veterinary supervision or oversight and those established as part of veterinary licensing and practice requirements and streamlining administrative procedures. To facilitate the transition from OTC to VFD status, FDA believes it is critically important that changes such as these be implemented to minimize impacts on veterinarians, the animal feed industry, and animal producers.

While FDA believes that all medically important antimicrobial new animal drug products should be marketed with the appropriate professional oversight restriction, at this time FDA is most concerned with medically important antimicrobial new animal drugs and combination new animal drug products intended for use in or on the feed or water of food-producing animals. As discussed in GFI#209, FDA's current methodology for assessing antimicrobial risks associated with the use of antimicrobial new animal drugs in food-producing animals is premised on the concept that increasing the exposure of bacterial populations to antimicrobial drugs increases the risk of generating resistance to those antimicrobial drugs. Because feed or water use antimicrobial drugs are typically administered to entire herds or flocks of food-producing animals, such uses pose higher risk to public health than the administration of such drugs to individual animals or targeted groups of animals. For that reason, this guidance is focused on those medically important antimicrobial new animal drugs that are approved for use in the feed or water of food-producing animals.

C. Additional Considerations

It is important to note that any extralabel use of medicated feed is not permitted by law (see sections 512(a)(2) and (a)(4)(A) of the FD&C Act). Neither veterinarians nor their clients may use, or direct the use of, a medicated feed in an extralabel manner. Therefore, when production claims for medically important antimicrobials are voluntarily removed from the approved labeling of these drugs, consistent with the judicious use principles of GFI #209, any further use of a drug without a production claim in medicated feed for production purposes will be considered an extralabel use and, thus, illegal.

V. Timeline for Voluntarily Implementing Changes

The Agency recognizes the significance of the proposed changes and the potential impacts such changes will have on the animal pharmaceutical industry, animal producers, the animal feed industry, and the veterinary profession. For this reason, FDA is currently pursuing a strategy for the voluntary adoption of these changes in an effort to minimize the impacts and provide for an orderly transition. FDA encourages all sponsors of affected new animal drugs and new animal drug combination products to contact the Agency and initiate steps to change product labeling and approved conditions of use through the process outlined in this guidance.

FDA also believes it is critical to see meaningful progress toward eliminating production uses of medically important antimicrobial drugs and bringing the remaining therapeutic uses of such drugs in or on the feed or water of food-producing animals under the oversight of veterinarians. In order to ensure progress under the cooperative framework outlined in this guidance, FDA will monitor progress to assess whether these changes are being adopted along the timelines discussed below. FDA is confident that the objective of phasing in these changes can be met through the cooperative process discussed in this guidance, which is why we are initially pursuing this voluntary approach. If, after the period of evaluation of the three year phase in, we determine that adequate progress has not been made, we will consider whether further action under the existing provisions of the FD&C Act may be appropriate. To assist FDA in effectively monitoring rates of adoption in the industry, we request that sponsors of affected products (i.e., those products containing antimicrobial new animal drugs of importance to human medicine that are administered in medicated feed or drinking water of food-producing animals) notify the Agency of their intentions to engage in the voluntary process to modify their product labeling within 3 months from the date of publication of this final guidance. FDA anticipates that sponsors of affected products should be able to complete implementation of the changes discussed in this final guidance within 3 years of the date of publication.

FDA intends to keep the public apprised of progress. First, FDA is making public on its website a listing of all antimicrobial products affected by the guidance. Second, FDA intends to notify affected drug sponsors and, following the 3-month notification period, FDA intends to publish summary information to provide an indicator of the level of engagement of affected drug sponsors in the voluntary process. In addition, the public will be notified of completed changes to affected products through publication of approval of supplemental new animal drug applications.

Upon issuance of this final guidance, the Agency will monitor the progress of its strategy for the voluntary adoption of the changes outlined, including the progress of measures intended to facilitate an orderly and minimally disruptive transition. Three years from the date of publication of this final guidance, FDA intends to evaluate the rate of adoption of the proposed changes across affected products. The Agency will then consider further action as warranted in accordance with existing provisions of the FD&C Act for addressing matters related to the safety of approved new animal drugs.

FDA recognizes that the proposed changes in the use of these antimicrobial drugs have significant practical implications for animal producers, veterinary practitioners, animal drug sponsors, and feed mills. In particular, as mentioned previously, implementing changes to streamline existing VFD requirements is pivotal to facilitating the transition to greater veterinary oversight (i.e., from OTC to VFD marketing status) for many of these products. Therefore, the 3-year timeframe for voluntary phase-in noted above is intended to provide sufficient time for the necessary changes to the existing VFD requirements to be developed and implemented through notice and comment rulemaking. Although FDA is committed to completing this rulemaking process within the 3-year timeframe for implementing the changes discussed in this guidance, FDA is prepared to extend the timeframe, as necessary, to ensure that it coincides with the implementation of the revised VFD requirements.

The 3-year timeframe for voluntary phase-in is also intended to provide time for animal drug sponsors to make these changes in an efficient and practical manner, and for other stakeholders to prepare for the resulting changes in management/business practices. When several approved products are involved (e.g., combination drug approvals containing the same active ingredients; same active ingredient in different dosage forms), sponsors are encouraged to coordinate implementation when practicable.

VI. Supplemental New Animal Drug Applications

A. Removing Production Uses/Changing Marketing Status

The procedures in this section (VI.A) apply to the situation where no new indications are being proposed. In the limited circumstances where a sponsor would be proposing that a new therapeutic indication be added, the procedures set forth at section VI.B below for submitting a supplemental application should be followed instead. As always, FDA encourages sponsors to consult with FDA prior to submitting supplemental applications to ensure that sponsors are targeting their submissions to answer questions that are relevant to the particular drug. The recommendations below, which, as guidance, establish no legally enforceable requirements, apply when sponsors who wish to voluntarily pursue judicious use changes are submitting supplemental new animal drug applications under 21 CFR 514.8.

1. Administrative Procedures

Sponsors who wish to voluntarily remove production use claims and change the marketing status for the remaining approved feed or water uses of affected products should indicate that their supplemental application is being submitted in accordance with GFI #213. Such supplemental applications do not need to include additional safety or effectiveness data. Sponsors of such applications would either (1) propose to change the marketing status to VFD or Rx and voluntarily withdraw the approval for all production uses or (2) for those applications without approved production uses, such sponsors would only propose a change in marketing status to VFD or Rx. No new indications would be proposed by the sponsors and in most cases the sponsors would only be required to submit revised labeling.

2. Applicable Supplemental New Animal Drug Application Technical Sections

Type A medicated articles and their associated medicated feeds should bear the VFD statement found in this Agency's regulations at 21 CFR 558.6(f) and medicated drinking water products (e.g., water soluble powders, concentrated solutions, etc.) should bear the Rx statement found in section 503(f)(4) of the FD&C Act (21 U.S.C. 353(f)(4)). The Type A medicated article and representative medicated feed labeling (Blue Bird) should be included in the supplemental application to verify: 1) the VFD statement found in this Agency's regulations at 21 CFR 558.6(f) has been appropriately added to all the labeling (Type A medicated article and Blue Bird feed labeling), and 2) the indications, mixing directions, feeding directions, etc., have been revised to reflect the voluntary withdrawal of the production use(s). Labeling for medicated drinking water products should be included in the supplemental application to verify: 1) the Rx statement found in section 503(f)(4) of the FD&C Act (21 U.S.C. 353(f)(4)) has been appropriately added to the labeling, and 2) the indications, directions for use, etc., have been revised to reflect the voluntary withdrawal of the production use(s).

B. Adding New Therapeutic Indications

In some cases, it has been suggested that there could be a therapeutic benefit associated with the production use of a drug. In situations where this could be the case, concerns have been raised that removing production uses from approved conditions of use will have negative animal health impacts. In those cases, where scientific evidence demonstrates a therapeutic benefit associated with the use of the drug for treating, controlling, or preventing a particular disease, sponsors could wish to seek new therapeutic indications to fill the therapeutic needs of animals.

FDA stresses that such new indications must be based on scientific evidence that such drug is safe and effective for the intended therapeutic use. Such new therapeutic indications should be directed at specifically identified diseases and should involve dosage regimens that provide the desired therapeutic effect while minimizing overall extent of use.

1. Administrative Procedures

Sponsors who wish to seek new therapeutic indications for use of affected products should indicate that their supplemental application is being submitted in accordance with GFI #213. Because new therapeutic indications are being proposed, these supplemental applications require the inclusion of additional safety and effectiveness data. These supplemental applications would need to include specific information as follows:

2. Applicable Supplemental New Animal Drug Application Technical Sections

a. Labeling

Type A medicated articles and their associated medicated feeds should bear the VFD statement found in this Agency's regulations at 21 CFR 558.6(f) and medicated drinking water products (e.g., water soluble powders, concentrated solutions, etc.) should bear the Rx statement found in section 503(f)(4) of the FD&C Act (21 U.S.C. 353(f)(4)). The Type A medicated article and representative medicated feed labeling (Blue Bird) should be included in the supplemental application to verify: 1) the VFD statement found in this Agency's regulations at 21 CFR 558.6(f) has been appropriately added to all the labeling (Type A medicated article and Blue Bird feed labeling), and 2) the indications, mixing directions, feeding directions, etc., have been revised to reflect the voluntary withdrawal of the production use(s). Labeling for medicated drinking water products should be included in the supplemental application to verify: 1) the Rx statement found in section 503(f)(4) of the FD&C Act (21 U.S.C. 353(f)(4)) has been appropriately added to the labeling, and 2) the indications, directions for use, etc., have been revised to reflect the voluntary withdrawal of the production use(s). In both cases, the labeling would need to reflect the new therapeutic indications for use.

b. Chemistry, Manufacturing, and Controls

The recommendations in this section assume there is no change in the chemistry, manufacturing and controls (CMC) information for the Type A medicated article or medicated drinking water products, including the product formulation, raw materials, manufacturing process, controls and packaging. If there are changes to the CMC information for the Type A medicated article or medicated drinking water product associated with the new therapeutic indication, the sponsor should provide a description of such changes in the supplemental application, along with appropriate documentation and data to support the changes. See 21 CFR 514.8(b).

Medicated Drinking Water Product

If the new indication provides for use of the medicated drinking water product at the same concentration or concentration range as currently approved, no additional chemistry, manufacturing and controls (CMC) information is required. If the medicated drinking water product will be used to prepare medicated water at a different concentration than currently approved, the sponsor should address stability of the medicated drinking water at the new concentration (Ref. 1).

Type A Medicated Article

If the new indication is for a currently approved species and provides for a medicated feed inclusion rate currently approved for that species, no additional CMC information is required.

If the new indication is for a medicated feed inclusion rate outside of the currently approved inclusion rate or range (i.e., lower than the lowest currently approved inclusion rate or higher than the highest currently approved inclusion rate for that species), the sponsor should address homogeneity, non-segregation, and stability of the drug in representative medicated feeds at the higher/lower inclusion rate (Ref. 1). In addition, the sponsor should demonstrate that the approved medicated feed assay method is valid for assay of feeds manufactured at the higher/lower inclusion rate or provide a new method that is capable of assaying the feed (Refs. 2, 3, and 4).

If the new indication is for a species not currently approved, the sponsor should address homogeneity, non-segregation, stability, and medicated feed assay methodology in representative medicated feeds at the highest and lowest proposed medicated feed inclusion rates.

c. Human Food Safety

Toxicology/Residue Chemistry

Toxicology information associated with the original approval was considered for currently approved antimicrobial new animal drugs, and that information was the basis of the acceptable daily intake (ADI) that drove the residue chemistry conclusions (target tissue, tolerance, withdrawal times, etc.) for those approvals. The toxicological assessment is not expected to be reconsidered under proposed therapeutic indications with similar conditions of use to those corresponding to the production use (see Impact on Human Intestinal Flora below). If a new, proposed therapeutic indication has corresponding conditions of use (same species, with dose/

duration/formulation/route of administration, etc.) that fit within existing residue chemistry parameters and are covered by previous residue chemistry evaluations, we do not anticipate that the sponsor will need to provide additional residue chemistry data or information. Sponsors are encouraged to contact CVM if they have any toxicological assessment questions.

Microbial Food Safety

Antimicrobial Resistance

It should be noted that, at the time of the original approval of older antimicrobial new animal drug applications, microbial food safety was most likely not considered in the same way or to the same extent as is currently the case. The Agency is concerned, consistent with the general elements of judicious use discussed in section II above and GFI#152, that giving antimicrobial drugs to food-producing animals at low levels for long periods of time and in large numbers of animals may contribute to antibiotic resistance. We expect any new indication(s) to (1) have an explicitly defined duration of dosing, (2) specify a therapeutic dose level, and (3) be available only to those animals that need the drug for the new indication, rather than the entire flock or herd when such use is not necessary.

Generally, these changes are expected to remove injudicious use indications, and to result only in the therapeutic use of medically important antimicrobial drugs in or on the feed or water of food-producing animals. In addition, such indications for use should include risk mitigation measures intended to reduce antimicrobial resistance when these drugs are used in or on the feed or water of food-producing animals.

To assure these goals have been met, the approval of any new indications for use would also necessitate that microbial food safety concerns be addressed consistent with the objectives of GFI #152. Prior to submission of an application, sponsors should discuss with CVM the type of information needed for this purpose. This information may include, but is not limited to:

1) Basic information on the subject antimicrobial new animal drug, including information on mechanisms of action, spectrum of activity, resistance mechanisms, transfer of resistance, pharmacokinetics and/or pharmacodynamics if known, proposed conditions of use and how these could influence resistance development, and information on susceptibility among bacteria of human health concern;
2) Information on the use of the subject antimicrobial new animal drug in or on the feed or water of food-producing animals, focusing on

numbers of animals treated, class, consumption rates for food products from treated animals, and rates of contamination by bacteria of human health importance.

3) Information on the use of the subject antimicrobial drug (or drugs similar to the subject drug) in human medicine. This information should address how loss of susceptibility of organisms of human health concern to the subject antimicrobial drug (or drugs similar to the subject drug) could impact human clinical medicine.
4) Information detailing how FDA's general elements of judicious use discussed in section II have been addressed. Specifically, all approved indications should be for treatment, control and/or preventive use only, require veterinary oversight, and restrict use to an explicitly defined duration of dosing. FDA considers these measures to be significant risk mitigations consistent with the goals of GFI #152.

Upon review of this information, the Agency should be able to: 1) identify appropriate risk mitigations that would enable us to determine that the proposed use of the drug in food-producing animals is safe (i.e., a reasonable certainty of no harm to human health); and 2) advise on the types of additional information or data needed to address any existing data gaps associated with the new, proposed use of the subject antimicrobial new animal drug.

Impact of Antimicrobial Residues on Human Intestinal Flora

Based on the expected changes in use patterns for new indications described in the previous section, we do not anticipate that this issue will need to be addressed by sponsors. However, if changes in conditions of use (dose/duration/formulation/route of administration) are proposed that are expected to increase overall human exposure to residues of antimicrobial new animal drugs in animal-derived food products, then sponsors will be asked to address the safety of their proposed use with respect to impact of residues or metabolites of antimicrobial new animal drugs and compounds with antimicrobial activity on the intestinal flora of human consumers (Ref. 5).

d. Target Animal Safety

Regarding previously approved antimicrobial new animal drugs, target animal safety information associated with the original approval has already been considered. As long as any new, proposed therapeutic indication has conditions of use that are covered by previous target animal safety evaluations (same species, a dose within the approved dosage range, same or shorter duration, same route of administration, same formulation), we do not anticipate that the sponsor will need to provide additional data or information, unless the Agency becomes aware of human or animal health concerns that were not apparent at the time of the original target animal safety evaluation.

e. Evidence of Effectiveness

Sponsors seeking approval of a new therapeutic indication should provide substantial evidence in support of the effectiveness of the new animal drug for the proposed new therapeutic indication. As described in 21 CFR 514.4, the sponsor should provide information that will allow the Agency to determine that:

- parameters selected for measurement and the measured responses reliably reflect effectiveness;
- the results obtained are likely to be repeatable;
- valid inferences can be drawn from these sources to the use of the new animal drug in the target population; and
- the new animal drug is effective for the new therapeutic indication under the proposed conditions of use.

The type of information required to demonstrate effectiveness will need to be determined on a case-by-case basis and be consistent with substantial evidence as described in 21 CFR 514.4. The Center will consider data from a wide variety of sources including literature, data generated by food animal production facilities or universities, and other existing information for a substantial evidence package. Sponsors should not limit their consideration of potential useful data to only data that is prospectively generated. Previously approved therapeutic indications that are very similar or "related" to the new therapeutic indication could also provide inferential value in support of the new indication (e.g., a new "control of bovine respiratory disease" indication added to an application that has a previously approved "treatment of bovine respiratory disease" indication with a similar dosage regimen).

Sponsors are encouraged to discuss approaches to satisfying the requirements of substantial evidence of effectiveness with CVM.

f. Environmental Impact

By regulation (see 21 CFR 514.1(b)(14)), the Environmental Impact section must include either an environmental assessment (EA) (see 21 CFR 25.40), or a claim for categorical exclusion (see 21 CFR 25.30, 25.33). Under

21 CFR 25.15(a), a claim of categorical exclusion must include a statement of compliance with the categorical exclusion criteria and must state that to the sponsor's knowledge, no extraordinary circumstances exist. "Environmental Impact Considerations" and directions for preparing an EA can be found in 21 CFR Part 25.

VII. Generic Drugs and Combinations

Revising the conditions of use in applications for a pioneer single ingredient new animal drug products may have an effect on abbreviated (generic) new animal drug applications and combination new animal drug applications that reference these single ingredient products. The effects that submission and approval of a supplement for the pioneer drug may have on these generic or combination drugs are discussed in this section. FDA intends to work expeditiously with the sponsors of affected generic and combination new animal drug applications to align their products with the revised conditions of use specified in the referenced (i.e., pioneer) applications for the single ingredient new animal drug products.

A. Generic Applications

If the approved conditions of use for a new animal drug application for a medically important antimicrobial new animal drug are revised under this guidance by voluntarily withdrawing a production use, the approved labeling for any currently approved generic application(s) that references the original new animal drug application must generally be revised in a similar fashion, as is now standard practice. FDA will contact affected generic drug sponsors when these revisions become necessary. Consistent with current practice, we expect that the generic sponsor will submit a supplemental application to come into compliance with the revised labeling of the reference listed new animal drug (RLNAD) within 60 days after FDA notifies the generic sponsor that the approved conditions of use for the RLNAD have been revised. In such cases, if the generic labeling is not revised accordingly, the generic application holder(s) faces the possibility of suspension of the generic application under section 512(c)(2)(G) of the FD&C Act (21 U.S.C. 360b(c)(2)(G)). With regard to suspension, FDA intends to follow the procedures outlined in its regulations at 21 CFR 314.153(b) relating to human generic drug suspensions until generic new animal drug regulations implementing section 512(c)(2)(G) of the FD&C Act (21 U.S.C. 360b(c)(2)(G) are finalized.

In addition, any future generic sponsor that wants to use such a drug as its referenced listed new animal drug cannot include the production use that was voluntarily withdrawn from the pioneer application in its generic application because under section 512(n)(1)(F) of the FD&C Act (21 U.S.C. 360b(n)(1)(F)) the generic sponsor must submit labeling that is the same as the labeling approved for the referenced listed new animal drug with a few exceptions not relevant here. Furthermore, under section 512(c)(2)(A)(vii) of the FD&C Act (21 U.S.C. 360(c)(2)(A)(vii)), the Agency cannot approve an abbreviated new animal drug application unless the labeling proposed for the generic product is the same as the labeling approved for the referenced listed new animal drug with a few exceptions not relevant for purposes of this draft guidance.

B. Combination New Animal Drugs

The term *Combination new animal drug* is defined in the substantial evidence provisions of 21 CFR Part 514 to mean a new animal drug that contains more than one active ingredient or an animal drug that is applied or administered simultaneously in a single dosage form or simultaneously in or on animal feed or drinking water (See 21 CFR 514.4(c)(1)(i)). Although the term combination new animal drug applies both to products intended for use in or on animal feed and products intended for use in the drinking water of animals, the majority of approved combination new animal drug products are feed use combination drug products.

Most feed use combination new animal drugs are combinations of individual Type A medicated articles that have previously been separately approved. So, for example, a 3-way feed use combination actually involves four approved new animal drug applications, one for the combination and one for each of the three individual Type A medicated articles. The holder of an approved feed use combination new animal drug application is typically also the holder of an approved application for at least one of the individual Type A medicated articles in the combination.

1. Production Uses

As discussed above, FDA is requesting affected sponsors to voluntarily withdraw production uses of their medically important antimicrobial new animal drugs and combination new animal drug products. In those instances where an approved combination new animal drug product with a production claim includes a medically important antimicrobial new animal drug and the sponsor of the individually approved new animal drug application for a medically important antimicrobial new animal drug has voluntarily withdrawn the production use claims, FDA expects the sponsor of the affected combination new animal drug product will voluntarily follow suit and similarly withdraw the production use claim from the combination new animal drug application. If sponsors of these affected combination new animal drug products do not voluntarily withdraw the production use claim from the combination new animal drug application, FDA intends to consider further action as warranted in accordance with existing provisions of the FD&C Act for addressing matters related to the safety of approved combination new animal drugs.

2. Remaining Therapeutic Uses

As discussed at section IV above, based on a number of factors FDA believes that the judicious use of medically important antimicrobial drugs intended for use in food-producing animals needs the scientific and clinical training of a licensed veterinarian. This belief applies not only to individual medically important antimicrobial new animal drugs but also to combination new animal drug products incorporating such drugs. However, as previously discussed, in recognition of the significant practical implications of revising the marketing status for these products, FDA has expressed its intent to pursue a strategy for voluntarily phasing in these changes over time in an effort to minimize the impacts and provide for an orderly transition. As explained more fully in section V, FDA is proposing clear timelines for sponsors of the affected products to make these changes in order to ensure effective progress under the cooperative framework outlined in this guidance.

However, once a sponsor of an individual Type A medicated article that is also part of a combination new animal drug submits a supplement to switch the marketing status of the individual product to VFD or Rx, FDA expects the sponsor of the affected combination new animal drug product to voluntarily follow suit. Indeed, for a combination new animal drug product containing individual Type A medicated articles intended for use in or on animal feed, this outcome is essentially compelled since a voluntary switch to VFD marketing status by one or more of the sponsors of the individual Type A medicated articles will automatically trigger the requirement for a VFD to be issued before the affected combination new animal drug product can be used in or on animal feed. This is the case because under section 504(a)(1) of the FD&C Act, "[a]ny animal feed bearing or containing a veterinary feed directive drug shall be fed to animals only by or upon a lawful veterinary feed directive issued by a licensed veterinarian in the course of the veterinarian's professional practice." (21 USC 354(a)(1)). Thus, the requirement for a VFD to be issued applies whenever a VFD drug will be used in feed, regardless of whether the VFD drug is being used by itself or in combination with other drugs. Because a voluntary switch to VFD marketing status by one or more of the Type A medicated articles contained in a combination new animal drug product results, by operation of law, in the requirement for a VFD to be issued before a feed containing the combination new animal drug product can be fed to animals, in effect, the combination new animal drug product takes on VFD status also.

Therefore, we believe that in such instances the combination new animal drug product sponsors should also submit their own supplements to formally change the marketing status of the affected combination new animal drug products to VFD in a timely manner.

This outcome is consistent with the Agency's policy, as expressed in the substantial evidence notice of proposed rulemaking (62 FR 59835; Nov. 5, 1997) which provides that a combination new animal drug should generally bear VFD or Rx marketing status if one or more of the new animal drugs that make up the combination product were individually approved with VFD or Rx marketing status for any of the intended uses or conditions of use that are also applicable to the combination product.

References

FDA 2008. Guidance for Industry 5: Drug Stability Guidelines.

FDA 2005. Guidance for Industry 135: Validation of Analytical Procedures for Type C Medicated Feeds.

FDA 2007. Guidance for Industry #136: Protocols for the Conduct of Method Transfer Studies for Type C Medicated Feed Assay Methods.

FDA 2007. Guidance for Industry #137: Analytical Methods Description for Type C Medicated Feeds.

FDA 2013. Guidance for Industry #159: Studies to Evaluate the Safety of Residues of Veterinary Drugs in Human Food: General Approach to Establish a Microbiological ADI VICH GL36(R).

FDA 2012. Guidance for Industry #209: The Judicious Use of Medically Important Antimicrobial Drugs in Food-Producing Animals.

In: Antibiotic Use in U.S. Livestock Production ISBN: 978-1-63485-056-8
Editor: Karin Greer

Chapter 4

ANTIMICROBIAL DRUG USE AND VETERINARY COSTS IN U.S. LIVESTOCK PRODUCTION*

Kenneth H. Mathews, Jr.

ABSTRACT

Antimicrobial drugs are fed to animals at low levels to treat diseases, to promote growth, and to increase feed efficiency. Incorporating low levels of antimicrobial drugs in livestock feeds has been shown to be a factor stimulating the development of antimicrobial drug-resistant bacteria in livestock. Since many of the drugs used to treat livestock are the same as or are related to drugs used in human health care, there is concern that resistant organisms may pass from animals to humans through the handling of animals or food derived from animals. The movement of pathogens from animals to humans, and vice versa, has been documented, but the extent to which it has occurred or could occur is unknown. Although it is estimated that as little as 10 percent of the problems of drug-resistant pathogens in humans originate in livestock health care practices, there is currently considerable debate about the frequency and costs of human disease outbreaks resulting from animals infected with drug-resistant pathogens. Several European countries have banned the

* This is an edited, reformatted and augmented version of Agriculture Information Bulletin 766, issued by the U.S. Department of Agriculture, Economic Research Service, May 2001.

growth-promoting use of antimicrobial drugs in livestock production as a precautionary measure to prevent resistant organisms from passing from animals to humans. This report presents preliminary estimates suggesting that discontinuing the use of antimicrobial drugs in hog production would initially decrease feed efficiency, raise feed costs, reduce production, and raise prices to consumers. Longer term effects were not examined.

Keywords: antimicrobial drugs, pathogens, growth promotion, feed efficiency, therapeutic drug use, subtherapeutic drug use, subclinical

INTRODUCTION

Antimicrobial drug resistance, the ability of bacteria or other microbes to resist the effects of antimicrobial drugs, is a global concern for both human health and agriculture (Swain Report to the English Parliament, the Institute of Medicine's National Research Council report (1980), the Council for Agricultural Science and Technology report, the Institute of Medicine report (1989), the World Health Organization report, the Committee on Drug Use in Food Animals report, and a General Accounting Office report). The specter of resistant livestock diseases affecting humans, human health, and human health care practices has heightened concerns about livestock drug use and motivated regulatory actions. In early 1999, the Center for Science in the Public Interest, representing 37 health and consumer groups, petitioned the U.S. Food and Drug Administration (FDA) to ban the use of penicillin, tetracycline, erythromycin, tylosin, lincomycin, virginiamycin, and bacitracin in livestock production (Reuters, March 9, 1999). A bill banning subtherapeutic feeding of the same seven antimicrobials was introduced into the House of Representatives in November 1999 (H.R. 3266, November 9, 1999). Several European countries have already banned the feeding of antimicrobial drugs to enhance growth or feed efficiency.

In the United States, the FDA has proposed a framework for evaluating and assuring the human safety of the antimicrobial effects of new animal drugs intended for use in food animals. The proposed guideline would classify antimicrobial drugs according to the extent to which they are useful in human health care. The new guidelines also propose setting predetermined thresholds for when actions should be taken to stem the emergence of resistant pathogens (Bernick).

The hypothesis that drug-resistant bacteria may be transferred to humans through food was first formally stated in 1969 (Swann). Proof of the actual transmission of antimicrobial-resistant diseases between animals and humans is difficult to establish and involves several steps: (1) the selection for and persistence of resistant bacteria in animals from subtherapeutic[1] doses of antimicrobial drugs, (2) the presence of resistant pathogens in animal products, (3) transmission of these pathogens to humans, and (4) diagnosis of human diseases caused by these pathogens (Cohen and Tauxe). In spite of the difficulties, studies tracing animal sources for human infection by drug-resistant pathogens do exist (Feinman; Holmberg, Wells, and Cohen; Okolo; Cohen and Tauxe; Lee et al.; and Thoen and Williams).

In animals, antimicrobial drugs are fed at low levels for therapeutic disease treatment or to promote animal growth and increase feed efficiency.[2] Walton points out that "a critical level or minimal inhibitory concentration (MIC) of antibiotic is needed to select resistance in bacteria" and that subtherapeutic levels to promote growth may not reach that critical level. However, correlations between drug-resistant bacteria and feeding practices using low levels of antimicrobial drugs are relatively high (Cohen and Tauxe; and Okolo).[3]

In humans, microbial resistance to antimicrobial drugs stems from over-reliance on antimicrobial drugs in human medicine, failure to adhere to prescriptions for the full duration of treatment, and increased clustering of people in hospitals, day care centers, and other similar places where humans congregate (*AHI Quarterly*). Two of the greatest sources of drug-resistant pathogens observed in humans are from drug-resistant pathogens encountered during hospitalization and misuse of antimicrobial drug prescriptions by both doctors and patients (U.S. Congress, Office of Technology Assessment and Committee on Drug Use in Food Animals). It is estimated that as little as 10 percent of the problems of antimicrobial resistance originate with livestock health practices (Bernick). The Committee on Drug Use in Food Animals offered the following perspective:

> "While the use of antibiotics in food animals can cause resistance emergence, not all instances of resistance are clinically significant, involve resistance in pathogens, or cause an actual illness. In contrast, because the occurrence of infection in hospitals is often considered life-threatening, the risk to human health of hospital-acquired infections might be thought of as a greater risk."

Other situations that motivate the evolution of drug-resistant microbes include essentially any long-term use of antimicrobial drugs in either animals or humans (Feinman; Holmberg, Wells, and Cohen; Okolo; and Cohen and Tauxe). Bans against using antimicrobial drugs in livestock production are often the first-mentioned line of defense against potential ineffectiveness of antimicrobial drugs in human health care.

This report explores these issues and presents background material on the economic importance of antimicrobial resistance and antimicrobial drug use in livestock production. The objectives of this report are to summarize previous estimates of economic effects of antimicrobial drug use and bans in livestock production and to present a simple thought experiment in which costs associated with the disuse of antimicrobial drugs in producing swine are estimated. Swine are affected by a large number of bacterial diseases, most swine receive subtherapeutic doses of antimicrobial drugs during the production process (USDA, APHIS and Hayes et al.), and a large proportion of swine are produced on large confinement operations where diseases can spread rapidly.

The ability of pathogens to move between humans and animals raises many questions. The extent to which this transfer can occur and has occurred is unknown (Figure 1). There is currently much debate about the frequency and costs of human disease outbreaks resulting from animals infected with antimicrobial drug-resistant pathogens. Food safety and human health depend in part on the production technologies employed to raise livestock, especially to the extent that pathogens or drug residues remain with the livestock all the way through the chain of processing events that begin at the farm and end with the consumer (Figure 2).

The economic consequences of resistance to antimicrobial and other drugs are difficult to measure precisely. Effects from resistant microbes and their associated costs can range from virtually no impact on animal health to costs that exceed the value of an animal.

The human health costs, while not addressed here, can also vary from no illness or discomfort to death.

Economic effects associated with low-level use of antimicrobial drugs in feeds may be negative, such as the possibility that costs of treating livestock diseases could be higher because of the necessity of using more expensive drugs effective on resistant pathogens.

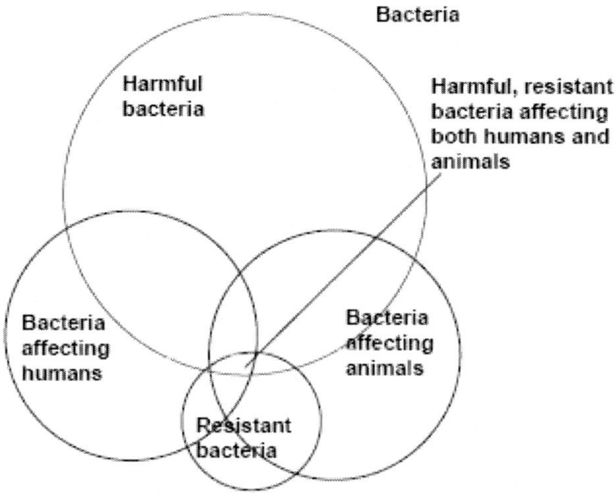

Figure 1. Universe of bacteria.

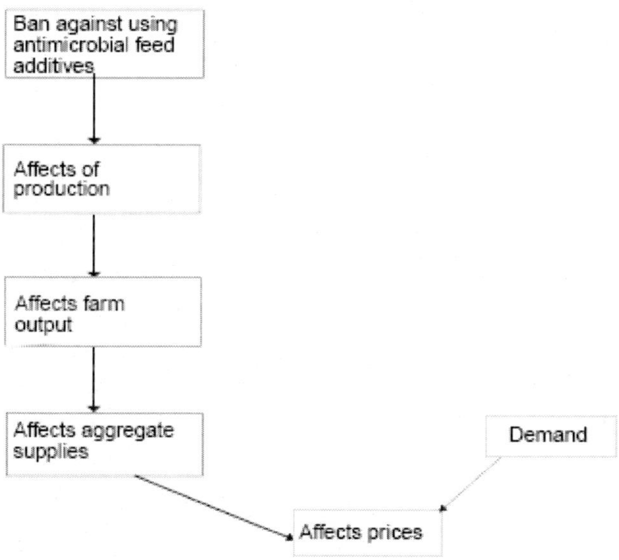

Figure 2. Effects of a ban on antimicrobials fed to livestock.

Or positive benefits could accrue to producers from not feeding low-level antimicrobial feed additives because of their ability to use less expensive antimicrobial drugs to treat disease outbreaks caused by susceptible pathogens. Benefits to consumers may, likewise, be positive, negative, or nonexistent.

Positive benefits could include livestock products without antimicrobial-resistant microbes and, thus, safer food. Or there may not be any benefits to consumers that would offset the higher costs from a ban.

The work described in this report contributes to the Economic Research Service's mission of providing economic analysis on efficiency, efficacy, and equity issues related to agriculture, food, the environment, and rural development to improve public and private decision making.

THE ECONOMICS OF USING DRUGS IN LIVESTOCK PRODUCTION

It is generally conceded that commercial livestock production in the United States, especially confinement production, would be virtually impossible without antimicrobial drugs. Therapeutic uses of antimicrobial drugs to treat specific infections can be at high or low levels. Although dosages below 200 grams per ton of feed are defined as subtherapeutic (Committee on Drug Use in Food Animals Panel on Animal Health, Food Safety, and Public Health), there may be no difference in the dosages for low-level therapeutic uses and uses of antimicrobial drugs as growth promotants—the only difference being the objective of drug administration.

In addition to therapeutic uses, antimicrobial drugs are fed to livestock for a variety of production management reasons. Low levels of antimicrobial drugs increase daily rates of weight gain and improve feed efficiency in livestock, lowering feed costs (Ensminger, 1987; North and Bell). Antimicrobial drugs in feed also slightly improve carcass quality in cattle (Ensminger, 1987). When steers and heifers are fed low levels of antimicrobial drugs, more fat is deposited and marbling increases, which can increase the value of the animal. When cattle are fed low levels of antimicrobial drugs, they have fewer diseases; therefore, fewer carcasses or livers are condemned during slaughter. Abscessed livers are particularly troublesome when feeding cattle rations containing relatively large amounts of grains and protein feeds. This occurs because antimicrobial drugs alter the microbial environment in the gastrointestinal tract, increasing the availability of some nutrients to the animal. Antimicrobial drugs can also alter metabolism of certain compounds, such as proteins and minerals, and can reduce stress from subclinical (a level of infection too low to produce noticeable symptoms) effects of pathogens. In either case, more energy contained in the feed is applied to growth and weight gain.

The effects of feeding low levels of antimicrobial drugs vary between livestock species. Rates of weight gain can be increased by about 6 percent and feed efficiency improved by about 4 percent in feeding beef steers and heifers for the slaughter market (Doane's). In swine, weight gains can be improved by about 10 percent and feed efficiency by about 5 percent (Doane's). Weight gains of up to 60 percent have been observed in dairy calves (Council for Agricultural Science and Technology (CAST)). Poultry growth and feed efficiency is also improved (North and Bell). Higher levels of production responses in swine have been reported in commercial settings than in experimental settings. The same pattern of higher commercial responses versus experimental responses likely persists for other livestock species. These improvements in production can amount to large economic gains for livestock producers.

In poultry production, especially broiler production, antimicrobial drugs are used as growth promotants in lieu of growth hormones for at least two reasons. First, no growth hormones are approved for use in poultry production. Second, hormones are ineffective in young birds because natural levels of hormones remain high for most of their relatively short production cycle.

Earlier committee, work group, and task force reports recommended banning subtherapeutic use of antimicrobial drugs in animal feeds as a precautionary response, despite insufficient evidence that human health problems arise directly from the practice (Swain Report to the English Parliament, the Institute of Medicine's National Research Council report (1980), the Council for Agricultural Science and Technology report, the Institute of Medicine report (1989), the World Health Organization report, the Committee on Drug Use in Food Animals report, and a General Accounting Office report). One author suggested that it is therapeutic uses that reach a critical level necessary for the development of resistant bacteria (Walton).

In most cases, however, therapeutic uses have been excluded from recommended bans.

A ban against using antimicrobial drugs in livestock production would come with a cost. Previous studies of the economic impacts of various partial and full bans of antimicrobial drugs in livestock feeds are summarized in Table 1. None of these studies addressed the effects of livestock drug bans on human health and health care. Results from earlier studies vary, but show higher costs to producers and generally price increases for consumers as the result of partial or total bans against feeding low levels of antimicrobial drugs to livestock (Table 1). Gilliam, et al.; Mann and Paulsen, and Wade and Barkley assumed a full ban of all antibiotics in feed; Dworkin and Headley looked at banning only selected antibiotics; and Allen and Burbee and USDA looked at both full and partial ban scenarios.[4] Gilliam et al., assumed a full ban on antimicrobial drugs and looked at three scenarios for fed cattle and hogs. They allowed production to remain constant by (1) lengthening feeding periods or (2) feeding more animals, or (3) allowing production to decline by feeding the same number of animals for the same period as without the bans. Gilliam et al. estimated consumer effects only for their third case in which production declined, translating the increased production costs into a price increase and transferring the entire increase to the consumer—a retail price increase of 7.18 cents per pound (1970 dollar equivalents). Allen and Burbee obtained similar results in a closely related study for broilers and turkeys looking at both full and partial antimicrobial bans with the same three production scenarios. Mann and Paulsen calculated producer and consumer effects of bans on antibiotics and DES (diethylstilbestrol) for five years after the bans. They found higher costs to producers and consumers. USDA looked at species by species bans on penicillin, tetracyclines, nitrofurans, and sulfas, a ban across all species, and economic effects for five years after bans with qualitatively similar results. They also estimated total and per capita costs incurred by consumers. Henson found increases in production costs under restrictions on adding penicillin, tetracyclines, and nitrofurans to poultry feed. Wade and Barkley found gains to both producers and consumers because of a ban on antibiotics used in pork production. The gain for consumers is due to their assumption that demand would shift outward because of increased pork consumption by health-conscious consumers. Their analysis focused on pork only, ignoring effects associated with other species. Hayes et al., also found increased costs to both producers, by about $6.05 initially, and consumers, by about $11 per family of four.

The authors of the CAST report included additional equilibrium price and quantity estimates based on price and quantity changes reported in several of the studies. The combined losses to producers and consumers ranged from just over a million dollars to $28 billion over a 5-year period. Losses were higher under the assumption of no substitutes for the antimicrobial drugs banned than under partial bans.

Table 1. Results from previous studies of full and partial bans against using antibiotic feed additives in livestock production

Study	Year study was published	Aggregate costs per year (million dollars)	Aggregate costs per year (results adjusted to 1998 dollars; million dollars)
Allen and Burbee; and Gilliam et al[1]	1972; 1973	5,660	12,707
Dworkin (Beef and pork only)[1]	1976	2,140	4,804
Mann and Paulsen[1]	1976	580	1,302
Headley[1]			
I (ban penicillin and tetracycline)	1978	1,440	3,233
II(ban nitrofuran and sulfa compounds)	1978	4,680	10,507
USDA II (moderate efficiency, penicillin, tetracyclines, sulfa drugs, and nitrofurans banned)[1]	1978	1,240	2,784
Wade and Barkley (4% decrease in Supply; Supply elasticity of 0.40; 5% increase in Demand;			
Demand elasticity of -2.50)			
Swine (loss in consumer surplus, 1987 dollars)	1992	11.74	16.85
Swine (loss in producer surplus, 1987 dollars)	1992	12.59	18.07
National Research Council/Institute of Medicine			
Partial ban	1998	1,261	1,281
Total ban	1998	2,527	2,566
Hayes et al.			
Losses to producers	1999	160.3	160.3
Losses to consumers	1999	748	748

[1]Data from Table 45 of the 1981 CAST report (Council for Agricultural Science and Technology, Antibiotics in Animal Feeds, Report No. 88): 5-year totals divided by 5 years.

Economic Considerations for the Animal Health Industry

The Animal Health Institute[5] (AHI) Resource Book states that one-third of the $2 billion spent on animal health products in 1992 was for commercial livestock. AHI estimates that about $600 million was spent on feed additives for all animals in the United States in 1992. Separately, the Office of Technology Assessment estimated that about 90 percent of the antimicrobial drugs used in agriculture are used as prophylactics or growth promotants. Applying this 90 percent to the AHI estimate of total dollars spent on animal health products suggest that about $667 million were spent on animal health products for commercial livestock in 1992, and about $600 million of this $667 million was for prophylactics and antimicrobial feed additives and $67 million for all other animal health products.

Veterinary Costs

Another way to estimate aggregate livestock health costs is to expand estimated costs per head from survey results. Per-head veterinary costs are available from Agricultural Resource Management Study (ARMS) data.[6] Estimates of total veterinary costs for livestock producers in 1998 were $0.39 per hundredweight (cwt) of milk produced (USDA, Agricultural Income and Finance Situation and Outlook), $1.15 per cwt gained for all hogs, $22.04 per bred beef cow, and 0.5 cent per pound of live broiler weight (Table 2). Expanding these costs per unit to represent total aggregate U.S. veterinary costs of production yields estimates on the order of $613 million for dairy, $747 million for beef cows and calves, $218 million for hogs, and $105 million for broilers. In addition to veterinary expenses, another $107 million was spent for antimicrobial feed additives for hogs in 1992 (Farm Costs and Returns Survey, unpublished information). There are additional classes of livestock, like sheep, goats, horses, rabbits, and others, for which there are either no estimates for or only sporadic estimates for drug costs or veterinary costs.

Table 2. Total veterinary costs for producing livestock, per unit and aggregate, 1998

Species/subgroup	Dollars per unit	Total millions dollars for U.S.
Beef cow/calf, all, per cow	22.04	746.83
Dairy, per cow, Milk, per cwt	.39	613.47
Hogs, all, per cwt gain	1.15	218.28
	Cents per pound	
Poultry, broilers, pounds live	.50	105.00

Sources: Beef cows, dairy, hogs (USDA, <http://www.ers.usda.gov/data/costsand returns/> (outdated web site)) and poultry (Christensen, 1993). Quantity data were from the USDA, Livestock, Dairy, and Poultry Situation and Outlook, LDP-M-68, February 29, 2000.

AN ESTIMATED AGGREGATE EFFECT OF NOT HAVING USED ANTIMICROBIAL DRUGS IN HOG PRODUCTION

Estimating the importance of antibiotic feed additives is significant in determining the impact of regulations or bans against feeding low levels of antibiotics to livestock. For instance, using the estimates for hogs from the foregoing, we can derive the following aggregate economic effects of feeding antibiotics and banning antibiotics.

Swine production easily ranks third in pounds of meat production behind poultry and beef, and is one of the top two livestock species in terms of antimicrobial drugs used at low levels in feed and water. In 1999, total hog production was 19.278 billion pounds (USDA 2000). To determine what effects feeding antimicrobial feed additives might have on livestock production, it is instructive to work through a basic economic assessment using assumptions about use of antimicrobial feed additives and associated feed efficiency. Assuming that a fourth of the 1999 hog production[7] was directly affected by antimicrobial feed supplements, including an improvement in feed efficiency of 5 percent, then antimicrobial feed supplements could have been directly responsible for 229 million pounds of the total 1999 U.S. hog production.

Total feed costs for all U.S. hogs were about $5 billion in 1999. Given a 1.25-percent improvement in feed efficiency from feeding low levels of antimicrobial drugs (the expected 5-percent improvement in feed efficiency applied to a fourth of total pork production), U.S. hog producers saved a total of about $63 million in feed costs.

This feed cost saving is offset by lost income from the effect of the additional hog production on hog prices. If hogs were the only commodity affected, and a supply and demand elasticities of .039 and -.48, respectively (Hahn), and assuming a supply shifter elasticity of 1.0 for hogs, the 229 million pounds of U.S. hog production lost had antimicrobial drugs not been fed would have resulted in prices about 2.3 percent higher than they were. That is, by feeding low levels of antimicrobial drugs, prices, at $34.02 per hundredweight (USDA, *Agricultural Outlook*) were $0.78 lower in 1999 than they might have been had antimicrobial drugs not been fed. A hypothetical reduction in hog production of 229 million fewer pounds from not feeding antimicrobial feed additives could have meant a price of $34.80 per cwt.[8] The lower production, about 19.049 billion pounds of total U.S. hog production had low-level antimicrobial drugs not been fed, would have been worth an extra $70 million.[9] Subtracting the extra feed costs ($63 million) from this $70 million leaves a net gain to the hog sector of $7 million. However, only $17.5 million, a fourth of the $70 million, would accrue to the producers who would have fed antimicrobial feed additives, but the entire extra feed cost of $63 million would have been theirs, leaving them with a net loss of $45.5 million.

If producers as a group are better off by not feeding antimicrobials to livestock, it seems natural to wonder why antimicrobial drugs are included in feed rations to improve growth rates and feed efficiency. The justification is a result of the large number of producers in the hog markets, each making optimal decisions about increasing production and efficiency, and each of which has no discernable effect in a competitive market. Each producer is able to improve his or her net returns by feeding antimicrobial drugs. However, when all producers act in concert, feeding antimicrobial drugs, the collective result is to increase hog supplies; the increased supplies decrease hog prices.

Several factors could mitigate results for the above thought experiment. First, it is not likely that an antimicrobial ban would only affect hogs. Drug use for beef, poultry, lamb, and fish would likely have been affected by a ban, and prices for those species would have been higher as well, because of less total meat available. Higher prices for other meat commodities would also reduce

Table 3. Antibiotic use on hog operations, December 1, 1994 through May 31,1995

Practice	Piglets Before or at Weaning	Market Hogs	Sows/ Gilts	Boars
	Percent of operations			
Antibiotics in feed	70.2	58.7	45.5	38.4
Antibiotics in water	16.0	12.3	6.6	4.7
Antibiotics injection	39.5	24.8	30.3	22.3

Source: Adapted from U.S. Dept. of Agriculture, Animal and Plant Health Inspection Service, Veterinary Services, Swine '95: Part I: References of 1995 Swine Management Practices, p. 12, October, 1995.

the effects on final consumption of hog price increases from a ban. Feed input prices for corn, sorghum, soybeans, cottonseed, and others would likely be higher because of increased demand for these and other inputs. These supply and price effects would likely decline as production adjusts over time due to increased production by producers who hadn't been feeding antimicrobial drugs and to adjusted production by other producers who had revised production practices previously dependent on low levels of antimicrobial drugs.

Second, not feeding the low levels of antimicrobial drugs in livestock feeds could contribute to increased production risks. Death losses and reduced production from diseases that had been prevented by feeding low levels of antimicrobial drugs could be costly. In situations where livestock are concentrated, especially in hog and poultry feeding operations, diseases can spread rapidly, and disease outbreaks can take a far heavier toll if low levels of antimicrobial drugs are not fed.

Toward Developing an Economic Model of Regulated Antimicrobial Use

The issues surrounding antimicrobial use are similar to issues surrounding other pest management and damage control problems. Other authors have recognized this similarity (Lichtenberg and Zilberman; Babcock, Lichtenberg, and Zilberman; and Fox and Weersink). Many of the regulatory issues raised in the context of animal drugs have been examined for pesticides and other agricultural chemicals (Carlson; Lazarus and Dixon; Harper and Zilberman; Zilberman et al.; and Zilberman and Millock). And some authors have specifically addressed the issue of the development of pesticide resistance (Hueth and Regev; Carlson; and Lazarus and Dixon).

Current antimicrobial drug use introduces several complexities into economic modeling of drug use in livestock production that are not characteristic of other pesticide-input use production models. First, low-level antimicrobial use in livestock production introduces additional complexities into the general pest management/pest resistance framework because feeding antimicrobial drugs at low levels is not only output-enhancing, but also is an input that interacts with other inputs, especially feeds.

Second, decision makers must consider tradeoffs between using and not using antimicrobial feed additives. Using antimicrobial feed additives yields productivity increases from growth and feed efficiency but increases the probability of a resistant disease outbreak and increases treatment costs due to using more expensive antimicrobial drugs to treat resistant diseases. Not using antimicrobial feed additives increases feed costs and perhaps costs associated with disease and death loss, but diseases are less likely to be caused by resistant pathogens and can often be treated with less expensive first-line antimicrobial drugs.

The welfare effects of antimicrobial feeding bans depend on assumptions about animal, producer, and consumer responses. Antimicrobial drugs are not yet part of any farm-level Hazard Analysis and Critical Control Point (HACCP) measures, but conceivably could become part of a regime to reduce pathogens at the farm level. To the extent feeding low levels of antimicrobial drugs to reduce food-borne pathogens became farm-level HACCP measures, welfare results could be complicated by conflicting policies to improve food safety and reduce antimicrobial drug use in livestock production.

IMPLICATIONS

The potential for antimicrobial drug-resistant pathogens to ultimately pass from animals to humans may increase with increasing levels of aggregate use of antimicrobial drugs. This is important to the extent these organisms are capable of causing disease or illness in humans. Incorporating low levels of antimicrobial drugs in livestock feeds is one factor stimulating the development of antimicrobial-resistant bacteria in livestock. Based on a precautionary principle, the practice of incorporating low levels of antimicrobial drugs in livestock feeds has been banned in some countries.

As incidents and problems involving drug-resistant pathogens increase, there will be more pressure for policies or regulations on using antimicrobial feed additives in U.S. livestock production. Economists and other scientists will be called upon to assess potential effects of these policies and regulations. Economic research in these areas of antimicrobial resistance and the use or nonuse of antimicrobial feed additives will depend on economic assessments of the effects of antimicrobial drugs in livestock feeds.

This analysis has presented a summary of literature on the economic effects of hypothetical antimicrobial bans and presented some preliminary estimates of the economic effects of using or not using antimicrobial drugs in swine feeding.

REFERENCES

AHI Quarterly 16 (3), *Animal Health Institute*, p. 4, Fall, 1995.

AHI Resource Book, *Animal Health Institute*, 1994-95.

Allen, G., and C. Burbee. "Economic Consequences of the Restricted Use of Antibiotics at Sub-Therapeutic Levels in Broiler and Turkey Production." (Mimeo) U.S. Department of Agriculture, Economics Research Service, Commodity Economics Division, 1972.

Babcock, B.A., E. Lichtenberg, and D. Zilberman. "Impact of Damage Control and Quality of Output: Estimating Pest Control Effectiveness." American *Journal of Agricultural Economics* 74: 163-72. 1992.

Bernick, J. "Resisting Resistance." *Dairy Today, Farm Journal*, Inc. Philadelphia, PA, March 1999.

Carlson, G.A. "Long-Run Productivity of Insecticides." *American Journal of Agricultural Economics* 59: 543-48. 1977.

Christensen, L.A. "Updating the ERS Broiler Cost and Returns Estimates." Livestock and Poultry Situation and Outlook. LPS-62, pp. 27-32. U.S. *Dept. of Agriculture, Economic Research Service*. Nov. 1993.

Cohen, M.L., and R.V. Tauxe. "Drug-Resistant Salmonella in the United States: An Epidemiologic Perspective." *Science* 234: 964-69. 1986.

Committee on Drug Use in Food Animals Panel on Animal Health, Food Safety, and Public Health, The Use of Drugs in Food Animals: Benefits and Risks. National Research Council, Board on Agriculture, and Institute of Medicine, Food and Nutrition Board, National Academy Press, Washington, DC, <<http://www.nap.edu/readingroom/>>July 28, 1998.

Council for Agricultural Science and Technology, Antibiotics in Animal Feeds, Report No. 88, Ames, IA, 1981.

Doane's Agricultural Report: Reference Volume. Doane's, 1988.

Dworkin, F.H. "Some Economic Consequences of Restricting the Subtherapeutic Use of Tetracyclines in Feedlot Cattle and Swine." (Mimeo) Office of Planning and Evaluation, Food and Drug Administration, OPE Study 33. 1976.

Ensminger, M.E. Dairy Cattle Science, Second Edition, *The Interstate Printers and Publishers*, Inc., Danville, IL, 1980.

Ensminger, M.E. Beef Cattle Science, Sixth Edition, *The Interstate Printers and Publishers*, Inc., Danville, IL, 1987.

Feinman, S.E. "The Transmission of Antibiotic-Resistant Bacteria to People and Animals." CRC Handbook Series in Zoonoses: Antibiotics, Sulfonamides, and Public Health. pp. 151-71. *CRC Press, Boca Raton*, FL. 1979.

Fox, G. and A. Weersink. "Damage Control and Increasing Returns." *American Journal of Agricultural Economics* 77: 33-9. 1995.

Gilliam, H.C., J.R. Martin, W.C. Bursch, and R.B. Smith. Economic Consequences of Banning the Use of Antibiotics at Subtherapeutic Levels in Livestock Production. Departmental Technical Report No. 73- 2, Department of Agricultural and Sociology, Texas A&M University, College Station, TX. September 1973.

Hahn, W.F. An Annotated Bibliography of Recent Elasticity and Flexibility Estimates for Meat and Livestock. U.S. Department of Agriculture, Economics Research Service, Commercial Agriculture Division, Staff Paper No. AGES-9611. 1996.

Harper, C.R., and D. Zilberman. "Pest Externalities from Agricultural Inputs." *American Journal of Agricultural Economics* 71: 692-702. 1989.

Hayes, D.J., H.H. Jensen, L. Backstrom, and J. Fabiosa. "Economic Impact of a Ban on the Use of Over-the-Counter Antibiotics." Staff Report 99 SR 90, Center for Agriculture and Rural Development, Iowa State University, Ames, IA. 1999.

Headley, J.C. Economic Aspects of Drug and Chemical Feed Additives. Unpublished background paper. Office of Technology Assessment, U.S. Congress, Washington, DC. 1978.

Henson, W.L. Economic Impact of Restriction on Use of Feed Additives in the Poultry Industry. A.E. and R.S. 147, Department of Agricultural

Economics and Rural Sociology, Agricultural Experiment Station, The Pennsylvania State University, University Park, PA, and U.S. Department of Agriculture, Economics and Statistics and Cooperative Service. 1980.

Holt, M.T., and S.R. Johnson. "Supply Dynamics in the U.S. Hog Industry." *Canadian Journal of Agricultural Economics* 36: 313-35. 1988.

Holmberg, S.D., J.G. Wells, and M.L. Cohen. "Animalto-Man Transmission of Antimicrobial-Resistant Salmonella: *Investigations of U.S. Outbreaks*, 1971- 1983." Science 225: 833-35. August, 1984.

Hueth, D., and U. Regev. "Optimal Agricultural Pest Management with Increasing Pest Resistance." *American Journal of Agricultural Economics* 56: 543-52. 1974.

Institute of Medicine, The Effects on Human Health of Antimicrobials in Animal Feeds, National Academy Press, Washington, DC, 1980.

Institute of Medicine, Human Health Risks with the Subtherapeutic Use of Penicillin or Tetracyclines in Animal Feed, National Academy Press, Washington, DC, 1989.

Lazarus, W.F., and B.L. Dixon. "Agricultural Pests as Common Property: Control of the Corn Rootworm." *American Journal of Agricultural Economics* 66: 456-65. 1984.

Lichtenberg, E., and D. Zilberman. "The Econometrics of Damage Control: Why Specification Matters." *American Journal of Agricultural Economics* 68: 261-73. 1986.

Mann, T., and A. Paulsen. "Economic Impact of Restricting Feed Additives in Livestock and Poultry Production." *American Journal of Agricultural Economics* 58: 47-53. 1976.

McBride, W.D., U.S. Hog Production Costs and Returns, 1992: An Economic Basebook. Rural Economy Division, Economic Research Service, U.S. Dept. of Agriculture, Agricultural Economic Report No. 724. Nov., 1995.

North, M.O., and D.D. Bell. Commercial Chicken Production Manual, Fourth Edition, Van Nostrand Reinhold, New York, NY, 1990.

Okolo, M.I.O. "Bacterial Drug Resistance in Meat Animals: A Review." International Journal of Zoonoses 13: 143-52. 1986.

Reuters, news release, March 9, 1999.

Shapouri, H., K.H. Mathews, Jr., and P. Bailey. Cow/Calf Costs of Production, 1990-91. Commodity Economics Division, Economic Research Service, U.S. *Dept. of Agriculture. Agriculture Information Bulletin* No. 670. June, 1993.

Swann, M.M. Report of Joint Committee on the Use of Antibiotics in Animal Husbandry and Veterinary Medicine. Cmnd. 4190. London: Her Majesty's Stationery Office. 1969.

Thoen, C.O., and D.E. Williams. "Tuberculosis, Tuberculoidoses, and Other Mycobacterial Infections." *In CRC Handbook of Zoonoses*, Ed. by G.W. Beran, pp. 41-59, CRC Press, Boca Raton, FL. 1994.

U.S. Congress, Office of Technology Assessment. Impacts of Antibiotic-Resistant Bacteria, OTA-H629 (Washington, DC Government Printing Office, Sept., 1995).

USDA, Agricultural Income and Finance Situation and Outlook. AIS-58, Rural Economy Division, Economic Research Service, Sept., 1995.

USDA, *Agricultural Outlook, Economic Research Service*, AGO-271, May 2000.

USDA, Animal and Plant Health Inspection Service, Veterinary Services. Swine '95: Part I: Reference of 1995 Swine Management Practices, Ft. Collins, CO, October, 1995.

USDA, Animal and Plant Health Inspection Service, Veterinary Services, Centers for Epidemiology and Animal Health, Antimicrobial Resistance Issues In Animal Agriculture <http://www.aphis.usda.gov/vs/ceah/cei/#antimicrobialresistance>, December, 1999.

USDA, Dairy Yearbook. Statistical Bulletin No. 924. Commercial Agriculture Division, Economic Research Service, 1995.

USDA, Economic Effects of a Prohibition on the Use of Selected Animal Drugs. Commercial Agriculture Division, Economic Research Service, 1978.

USDA, Poultry Yearbook. Statistical Bulletin No. 916. Commercial Agriculture Division, Economic Research Service, *Agricultural Economic Report No. 414*. 1994.

USDA, Livestock, Dairy, and Poultry Situation and Outlook, LDP-M-68, Market and Trade Economics Division, Economic Research Service, February 29, 2000.

USDA, http://www.econ.ag.gov/briefing/farmincome/car/ Resource Economics Division, Economic Research Service, March 28, 2000.

U.S. General Accounting Office, Food Safety: The Agricultural Use of Antibiotics and Its Implications for Human Health. GAO/RCED-99-74. 1999.

Wade, M.A., and A.P. Barkley. "The Economic Impacts of a Ban on Subtherapeutic Antibiotics in Swine Production." *Agribusiness* 8: 93-107. 1992.

Walton, J.R. "Impact of Antibiotic Restrictions in Animal Production on Public Health." *Journal of Animal Science* 62: 74-85. 1986.

World Health Organization. The Medical Impact of the Use of Antimicrobials in Food Animals: report of a WHO meeting, Document No. WHO/EMC/ZOO/97.4, Berlin, Germany, 1997.

Zilberman, D., A. Schmitz, G. Caterline, E. Lichtenberg, J.B. Siebert. "The Economics of Pesticide Use and Regulation." *Science* 253: 518 - 22. 1991.

Zilberman, D., and K. Millock. "Pesticide Use and Regulation: Making Economic Sense Out of an Externality and Regulation Nightmare." *Journal of Agricultural and Resource Economics* 22: 321-32. 1997.

End Notes

[1] Subtherapeutic doses of antimicrobial drugs were generally considered to be less than 50 grams of antimicrobial per ton of feed for these studies. More recently, subtherapeutic doses are considered to be less than 200 grams per ton of feed.

[2] Growth rate is defined as pounds of weight gained per day. Feed efficiency is defined as pounds of feed fed per pound of gain. The two measures are related, but not identical: A 2-pound-per-day rate of gain (growth rate) can be achieved by feeding different amounts of even the same feed to different animals. And different animals can gain a pound on the same amount of feed (feed efficiency) but gain different amounts per day.

[3] For a collection of recent papers on selected aspects of the biology of antimicrobial drug resistance in livestock production, see the report by the U.S. Department of Agriculture's Animal and Plant Health Inspection Service (APHIS), Antimicrobial Resistance Issues In Animal Agriculture, <http://www.aphis.usda.gov/vs/ ceah/cei/#antimicrobial resistance>.

[4] The Allen and Burbee (1972), Dworkin (1976), and Headley (1978) papers were not reviewed by this author, but their studies were summarized second-hand from reviews in the CAST report (1981).

[6] The Agricultural Resource Management Study (ARMS) is described on the web site listed in the References section under USDA, 2000.

[7] The assumption that a fourth of hog production was directly affected by feeding antimicrobials is conservative in view of the shares of operations feeding antimicrobials observed in APHIS data included in Table 3.

[8] These results assume that the same number of hogs would have been fed the same amount of feed as was the case, but these hogs would have reached slightly lower slaughter weights because of the loss in growth and feed efficiency. It may be that producers would simply continue to feed their hogs to the same market weights, in which case, results of this thought experiment would be slightly different quantitatively, but not qualitatively.

[9] 19.278 billion pounds of hog production at 34.02 per hundredweight was worth about $6.56 billion; 19.049 billion pounds at the higher price (price and quantity are inversely related) of $34.80 was worth $6.63 billion, $70 million more. This result derives from the effects of low commodity elasticities common in agriculture on total values.

INDEX

A

B

C

I

J

L

M

N

O

P

Q

R